UNDERSTANDING THE **SOCIOLOGY** OF **HEALTH**

AN INTRODUCTION

SECOND EDITION

ANNE-MARIE BARRY AND CHRIS YUILL

companion website ↖

SAGE Publications
Los Angeles ▪ London ▪ New Delhi ▪ Singapore

First edition published 2002
Reprinted 2003
This second edition published 2008

SAGE Publications Ltd
1 Oliver's Yard
55 City Road
London EC1Y 1SP

SAGE Publications Inc.
2455 Teller Road
Thousand Oaks, California 91320

SAGE Publications India Pvt Ltd
B 1/I 1 Mohan Cooperative Industrial Area
Mathura Road
New Delhi 110 044

SAGE Publications Asia-Pacific Pte Ltd
33 Pekin Street #02-01
Far East Square
Singapore 048763

Library of Congress Control Number: 2007928800

British Library Cataloguing in Publication data

A catalogue record for this book is available from the British Library

ISBN 978-1-4129-3622-4
ISBN 978-1-4129-3623-1 (pbk)

Typeset by C&M Digitals (P) Ltd., Chennai, India
Printed and bound in Great Britain by TJ International Ltd, Padstow, Cornwall
Printed on paper from sustainable resources

In memory and celebration of

Mike Hepworth

Scholar, gentleman and all round good guy

Contents

Acknowledgements

We would like to thank Julian Bell for his help and support in creating that most valuable of all entities (time!) to engage in this project. Special mention must also be made of Emmanuelle Tulle, Lydia Lewis, Val Sheach-Leith, Donncha Marron and June Wells for their help and advice. Their contributions greatly assisted the completion of this book, but as always, any shortcomings are ours and not theirs!

This whole project would not have reached completion without the support of Natalie Aguilera at Sage and the anonymous referees who have commented on various drafts at various stages.

A big thank-you is also in order for all the Health Sciences students at Robert Gordon University who have helped enormously in providing feedback and ideas on how to communicate sociology to people encountering it for the first time.

Chris would also like to thank the janitors at Robert Gordon University for their conversation during the late nights and weekends that went into writing this book, as well as the staff at Rock, Salt and Nails and At The Arches for their damn fine coffee.

Anne-Marie would like to thank Aidan for being such a wonderful son.

Finally, must mention everyone who enjoyed that little 'Sunshine on Leith' on a snowy day in Glasgow in 2007!

Guided tour

1

Sociological theory: explaining and theorising

MAIN POINTS

* Sociology is a scientific approach to understanding people in society.
* Social structures can often exert more influence over our behaviour than we would expect.
* Sociological perspectives on health emphasise that it is vital to understand the social in order to fully understand health and illness.
* The sociological imagination invites us to think beyond our own subjective perceptions.
* Sociological theories are useful in moving away from commonsense understandings of society.

KEY CONCEPTS

The sociological imagination, structure, agency, theory, discourse functionalism, symbolic interactionism, Marxism, feminism, discourse and postmodernism.

Main Points: An outline of the important points and conclusions that will be discussed in depth throughout the chapter.

Key Concepts: A useful and quick guide as to which concepts are going to be discussed in the chapter to come.

Introduction

The aim of this chapter is to introduce the discipline of **sociology** and to focus, in particular, on the significance of the sociological study of health, illness and medicine for health-related professions. In order to do so it is necessary to begin by establishing the scope and remit of sociology as a subject area *and* as an explanatory method.

Sociology is concerned with the study of **society** and specifically with key issues such as explaining change and the distribution of power between different social groups. The discipline of sociology also offers its students specific methods of investigation and explanation. For example, this chapter introduces you to the concept of the **sociological imagination**, asking you to adopt a critical and questioning approach to even the most mundane aspects of social life. Sociological knowledge is based on a 'scientific' approach built upon evidence to support theoretical perspectives. This chapter offers an introduction to a range of sociological perspectives.

1.1   Sociology: a method of enquiry and explanation

Sociology is the study of the interaction between groups and individuals in human society. The term **society** refers to a range of external factors that influence our beliefs and behaviours.

The raw material of sociology is human society, the development of groups, and the ways in which social groups are organised and change over time. Sociology is, therefore, the study of society. Such a statement, however, tells us very little about sociology and does nothing to draw out what is distinctive about the discipline in relation, for example, to psychology or simply to our own observations of society and social groups. Sociology is concerned with the study of human society (Giddens 1994: 7) in terms of the interaction between individuals and groups and the interaction between groups. It is not individuals, *per se*, who draw our attention, but how they interact with the social environment. Giddens uses the term society to refer to 'a cluster, or system of institutionalised modes of conduct' (Giddens 1997: 7). Sociologists refer to society as a 'system' and our own behaviour as 'institutionalised' to draw attention to what is external to the individual, that is 'society' itself. 'Society' refers to the structural or external factors that influence our beliefs and behaviour and that establish some predictability and regularity in our lives.

What troubles many new students of sociology is the suggestion that something referred to as 'society' shapes or determines our behaviour. Such an explanation seems to take away what is individual about us and suggests that our behaviour and

Introduction: Sets the scene as to what will be discussed and reviewed in the forthcoming chapter.

Marginal Definitions: A useful, accessible and easy-to-find definition of a concept or theory that has been mentioned in the main text.

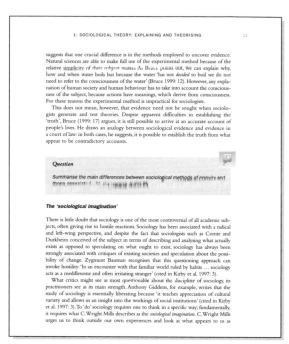

Questions: Prompts to assist in the understanding and contemplation of important points and issues raised in the text.

Links: Indicate where more in-depth or complementary information about a certain topic can be found elsewhere in the book.

Examples: Assist in the understanding of concepts and theories by providing practical and 'real-life' illustrations of what the concept or theory attempts to understand.

Conclusion: Pulls together and discusses the main points of a chapter while offering some observations on how they further illuminate an understanding of health from a sociological perspective.

Summary Points: All the main issues and points that have been raised and discussed in the chapter are brought together in one succinct section.

Case Study with Discussion Questions: A vignette of an individual that acts as an exemplar of the issues discussed in the chapter with questions that assist in the focussing and application of the various theories and concepts that have been discussed.

Taking Your Studies Further: After reading the chapter, various suggestions – in the form of journal articles, books and websites – are offered to assist in gaining more in-depth and detailed knowledge that goes beyond an introductory level.

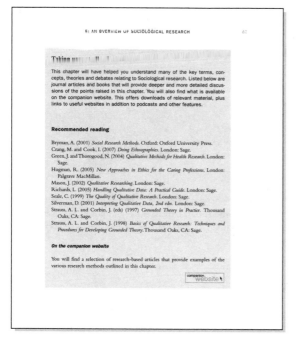

Recommended Reading: Suggestions for other readings that provide deeper and more detailed information on the issues raised in the chapter.

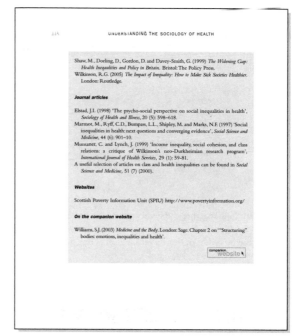

On the Companion Website: Indicates further material can be found on the website including podcasts, links to other websites, downloadable journal articles and book chapters.

Companion website

Visit the companion website at xxx to find a range of teaching and learning material for lecturers and students including the following:

For lecturers:

- Tutors' notes: This is a useful resource for the busy or new lecturer and sets out chapter-by-chapter seminar guides. Each seminar relates to the main points in the chapter and has suggestions for reading, useful web links, student activities and discussion points.
- PowerPoint slides: In addition to the notes, each chapter has its own dedicated PowerPoint slide show. The slides relate to the main points of the chapter and can be used as they are or adapted to meet lecturers' particular needs.

For students:

- Downloadable journal articles: Once you have read through the chapter and gained a good knowledge of the basics of a particular issue you can take your studies further by accessing a more in-depth and detailed scholarly article.
- Relevant web links: The internet provides a bewildering range of material and resources, here you can go straight to a website that is both scholarly sound and complements the material in the chapter.
- Online glossary: Sociology can often present new concepts and ideas that can be a little daunting to grasp at first. This resource provides a useful and accessible collection of those key concepts and terms.
- Podcasts: This feature will offer a range of ten-minute podcasts that will cover a particular topic, concept or issue. Ideal for engaging in the material when not in a university or college context.

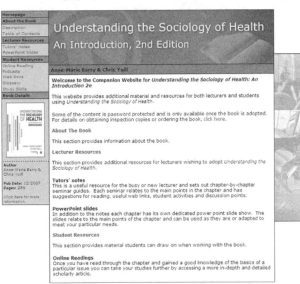

Introduction

How to use this book

First of all, it is best not to think of this solely as a book. What you have before you is just one part of an array of media to assist in an introduction to sociological perspectives on health and illness. There are other resources to be found on the companion website that allow you to, for example, read more deeply into the topics presented in this book with access to chapters from more advanced publications or whole journal articles. Additionally, further resources also allow you to approach the issues using other formats such as websites or podcasts. To maximise what we are offering, you should both sign up to the website and check for updates and new material on a regular basis. There will also be facilities for contacting us, the authors, to put forward your ideas on what is useful and not so useful about what we have provided.

This book will, however, be the main starting point for your studies and we shall say a little more about it now. As with any introductory text, we have to be selective in what is covered and in what depth. It is written with the assumption that most people who are using this book have had little prior contact with sociology and are unfamiliar with what sociology seeks to do and how it explores and makes sense of health and illness. With that in mind, we have chosen to highlight what we see as the main issues and debates within the sociology of health and illness and to try to put them across as clearly as possible. This means adopting what we hope is an accessible prose style that does not lapse into an unnecessarily complex academic mode or become too conversational. We have also chosen not to use too many references within the actual text in order to assist clarity. References to further reading are available at the end of every chapter and on the companion website.

Throughout the book you will see various features, both in the margins and embedded in text, which will offer one of the following three facilities. *Definitions*: the meanings of key concepts and technical expressions are summarised here. *Questions*: prompts to provide reflection and discussion of the points raised in the text. *Links*: indications of where complementary and further information can be found.

The book falls into three sections. The first section ***Theories, Perspectives and Concepts*** (Chapters 1–5) provides an overview of sociological perspectives on health and how we begin to research and understand society. This begins in Chapter 1 by defining and exploring sociology, sociological theory and the sociological imagination. We then move on, in Chapters 2-4, to interrogate medicine as the dominant mode of understanding health. This takes in tracing the roots of medicine during the Enlightenment and the particular discourse of health that it offers. Attention then turns in Chapter 5 to how sociology attempts to understand health and the variety of approaches and methods that sociologists use in their research.

The second section *Key Themes* (Chapters 6–11) deals with the main health inequalities of class, 'race' and gender along with mental health, the body and ageing. It is here that the main social processes and structures that influence, shape and pattern health, the body and illness will be investigated. What will become evident is that the power that society exerts is often more influential on our health than our own decisions and choices. For example, we will review how issues such as poverty and racism negatively impact on the health of a wide variety of people.

The final section, *Contexts* (Chapters 12–13) examines the wider influences, issues and social policies relating to the provision of institutional or community care. Here, we shall appraise the changes that have occurred in the area of health and social care provision and how subsequent policy moves have seen an increasing emphasis on the community as a place of care.

SECTION 1

Theories, Perspectives
and Concepts

1

Sociological theory: explaining and theorising

MAIN POINTS

- Sociology is a scientific approach to understanding people in society.
- Social structures can often exert more influence over our behaviour than we would expect.
- Sociological perspectives on health emphasise that it is vital to understand the social in order to fully understand health and illness.
- The sociological imagination invites us to think beyond our own subjective perceptions.
- Sociological theories are useful in moving away from commonsense understandings of society.

KEY CONCEPTS

The sociological imagination, structure, agency, theory, discourse functionalism, symbolic interactionism, Marxism, feminism, discourse and postmodernism.

Introduction

The aim of this chapter is to introduce the discipline of **sociology** and to focus, in particular, on the significance of the sociological study of health, illness and medicine for health-related professions. In order to do so it is necessary to begin by establishing the scope and remit of sociology as a subject area *and* as an explanatory method.

Sociology is concerned with the study of **society** and specifically with key issues such as explaining change and the distribution of power between different social groups. The discipline of sociology also offers its students specific methods of investigation and explanation. For example, this chapter introduces you to the concept of the **sociological imagination**, asking you to adopt a critical and questioning approach to even the most mundane aspects of social life. Sociological knowledge is based on a 'scientific' approach built upon evidence to support theoretical perspectives. This chapter offers an introduction to a range of sociological perspectives.

1.1   Sociology: a method of enquiry and explanation

Sociology is the study of the interaction between groups and individuals in human society. The term **society** refers to a range of external factors that influence our beliefs and behaviours.

The raw material of sociology is human society, the development of groups, and the ways in which social groups are organised and change over time. Sociology is, therefore, the study of society. Such a statement, however, tells us very little about sociology and does nothing to draw out what is distinctive about the discipline in relation, for example, to psychology or simply to our own observations of society and social groups. Sociology is concerned with the study of human society (Giddens 1994: 7) in terms of the interaction between individuals and groups and the interaction between groups. It is not individuals, *per se*, who draw our attention, but how they interact with the social environment. Giddens uses the term society to refer to 'a cluster, or system of institutionalised modes of conduct' (Giddens 1997: 7). Sociologists refer to society as a 'system' and our own behaviour as 'institutionalised' to draw attention to what is external to the individual, that is 'society' itself. 'Society' refers to the structural or external factors that influence our beliefs and behaviour and that establish some predictability and regularity in our lives.

What troubles many new students of sociology is the suggestion that something referred to as 'society' shapes or determines our behaviour. Such an explanation seems to take away what is individual about us and suggests that our behaviour and our beliefs are not unique but may be determined by an external force and replicated by many other individuals. On reflection, however, this process of shaping and influencing is evident in all that we do. **Socialisation** into the norms and values of a particular society enables us to predict and make sense of the behaviour of others and ourselves. 'Society' provides us with the cultural resources to live in the social world because patterns of behaviour, responses and ways of behaving are not invented anew each day but exist outside any one individual. In most human encounters within a specific society, there are roles to be played out, responses that can be predicted and cues that are acted upon.

Socialisation refers to the process whereby we become aware of the values and beliefs of society.

Question

Pause for a moment and ask yourself how many of our own actions and responses are automatic in the sense that we 'know' how to act in that given situation.

Rosenhan's study, 'On being sane in insane places' (1973), is an excellent illustration of the potential for our identities to be imposed on us by others. Rosenhan's experiment involved eight researchers posing as 'insane' who presented themselves to mental health professionals, claiming to hear voices. Apart from the supposed symptoms, the researchers told the truth about their circumstances and background. All eight researchers were admitted to hospital. Except for the initial alleged symptoms, the researchers acted normally and upon admittance stated that they no longer had any symptoms. According to Rosenhan, it is therefore problematic to say that we 'know' what insanity is. The medical professionals in this case responded to certain cues (alleged symptoms) and interpreted the researchers' behaviour and histories in the light of their assumed insanity. This experiment is important in so far as it illustrates the way in which others can impose identities upon us. The behaviour of the researchers was interpreted in the light of a set of shared symbols and meanings. In this case, the shared symbols and meanings referred to the diagnostic categories developed and used by the medical profession. The diagnosis of insanity only had meaning in the light of these categories. This particular experience begs the question of whether patients actually present 'real' symptoms or whether the symptoms are in the minds of the people who make the diagnosis.

A further example of the way and extent to which the group influences individual behaviour can be illustrated with reference to the work of Festinger et al.

(1956). In this case, the group was a cult that was prophesying the end of the world by a very specific date and time. When the prophecy was proven false, the beliefs of the group members were *not* fundamentally altered. A message from God, relayed by the group leader, indicated that the end of the world was not to happen at this point after all, since the group manifested such goodness that the world would be saved from destruction. Festinger then asks why beliefs persist even in the light of contradictory evidence. The explanation lies within the group itself and its ability to reinforce the original belief. The power to do so is greater when the group consists of a close network without any dissenters. Festinger notes that, in this case, people who had been part of the group but who had not gathered in one place prior to the alleged catastrophe did not show the same adherence to the original prophecy.

Links

Chapter 6 provides an example of the complex relationship between structural factors and personal choice in relation to health inequalities.

The relationship between society and individuals

Thus far this discussion has been concerned to demonstrate what sociology 'is' by examining the subject matter or what has been referred to as the 'raw material' of study, namely society. However, the discussion has developed further in terms of suggesting a specific and distinct relationship between individuals and the society or **'structure'** in which they live. A helpful example of the way in which structure (society) influences the actions and experiences of individuals is provided by Giddens. He uses the analogy of language to illustrate the relationship that individuals have with the wider social structure. None of us has invented the language that we use but without it social activity would be impossible because it is our shared meanings that sustain 'society'. However, as Giddens (1994) also points out, each of us is capable of using that language in a creative, distinct and individual way, and yet no one person creates language. In the same way human behaviour is not determined in a mechanical way by the structure we call society. Later chapters discuss the significance of social **class** in determining levels of morbidity and mortality and yet not every person in each social class category will have identical experiences. There will, however, be enough similarities in patterns of health within each social class for us to justifiably place people in these specific groupings. Similarities in people's experiences can be seen in terms of income levels, of availability of local resources such as GPs, of geographical location, and of their physical environment and patterns of expenditure. The relationship and interplay between society and the individual is explained in terms of **structure** and **agency**. The latter is a concept used to refer to a cluster of ideas about the potential for individuals to determine their lives, to change their environment and, ultimately, to influence the wider structure. The concept of agency, therefore, allows us to appreciate the way in which we are shaped by society, and in turn shape society.

If the subject matter of sociology is human society, and behaviour is explained primarily in terms of 'structure', then this logically denotes specific factors in the explanatory framework of the discipline. Sociological explanations of what determines our state of health will necessarily differ from, for example, biological explanations. Clearly disease is a biological and physical entity experienced through the medium of the body. The causes of disease, while biological, can also be considered in terms of social and structural factors. The immediate cause of a disease may be infection but the factors that lead to this may be many and varied. If we reflect upon patterns of morbidity and mortality over the last two centuries, then it is possible to observe a significant shift away from infectious diseases to chronic conditions. Commentators such as Doyal (1979) argue that improved standards of living, better hygiene and the availability of medicine via the NHS have caused this change. In other words, when we consider the factors that influence a person's state of health, the risk of infection, an ability to fight infection and genetic predisposition are greatly important but, within sociology, these are not our main focus. Social and environmental factors such as age, social class and **gender** are as, if not more, important.

The term **structure** is similar to that of 'society' in so far as it draws our attention to those factors that help determine our experiences through the establishment of expected ways of behaving. In contrast, the concept of **agency** reminds us that individuals do not simply act out predetermined roles but 'interpret'. those roles in a way unique to them.

Question

Gender is a good example of how structures shape our lives and how we make individual choices about how we live. In your experience as a man or woman, what experiences do you share in common with your gender? In what do you consider yourself 'unique' and different from all other women or men?

A **sociological understanding of health** considers structural and social factors, rather than simply biological explanations of health and disease.

It is possible to define what we mean by 'sociology' by sketching out the discipline's remit in terms of the study of human society. From this it is logical to conclude that the study of sociology is relevant to understanding and explaining health in so far as health

In historical terms, **modern** is a term used to refer to the time period from the late nineteenth century to the mid-twentieth century.

and its determinants need to be explained within a social context. Within nurse education, for example, the emphasis placed on 'holistic' care can also be used to justify the study of sociology in that it provides information that places an individual within a social context. To conclude that this is all that the discipline of sociology can offer in terms of studying health, illness and medicine is mistaken and unnecessarily limiting. What sociology offers is a questioning and critical way of thinking and a distinct **method** of explanation. To fully appreciate this element of sociology it is helpful to understand, how, why and when the discipline came into being.

The historical origins of sociology

The discipline of sociology is fundamentally a 'modern' one, bound up with attempts to explain, anticipate and alter a rapidly changing world. According to Giddens (1997: 5), the focus of sociology at its inception was the structures and relationships that derived from industrialisation (Giddens 1997: 7). An examination of the works of the founding fathers of sociology (Comte, Durkheim, Weber and Marx) suggests a preoccupation with attempts to understand a rapidly changing world and to do so in a way that was 'scientific', objective and rational. Auguste Comte, for example, believed that the development of any society was ultimately positive and progressive, and identified three different phases: the religious, the metaphysical and the scientific. Each of these phases represented a mode of thought and explanation: the religious period represented a supernatural interpretation of the world, the metaphysical one replaced religion with a belief in forces such as nature, and the final, scientific, stage represented the most positive and rational phase of human development (Craib 1997: 23). Understanding this new and complex society meant adherence to rational, scientific and empirical methods. The underlying motivation of the discipline was to reveal the reality of social relationships. For Karl Marx, this meant making plain the 'real' relationships of power and exploitation behind social class. For Emile Durkheim, getting to the heart of the reality meant the observation and recording of 'facts' to provide a picture of the world as it is, rather than to anticipate how the world should be.

Sociology strives to be 'scientific' in the sense that it seeks to evidence its findings and to ensure that explanations are consistent. A fundamental difference between the social and natural sciences is that the subject matter of the social sciences, unlike that of the natural sciences, is human beings and their behaviour.

Can sociology be 'scientific'?

To the extent that sociological explanations attempt to be rational and empirical they share certain features with scientific disciplines. According to Bruce (1999), scientific explanations are consistent (that is to say they cannot contradict themselves), they must accord with the evidence, and when evidence is found to refute the explanation, the explanation itself must be changed (Bruce 1999: 3). A fundamental issue for sociologists is whether sociology is a science in the same sense as the physical sciences. Bruce suggests that one crucial difference is in the methods employed to uncover evidence. Natural sciences are able to make full use of the experimental method because of the relative simplicity of their subject matter. As Bruce points out, we can explain why, how and when water boils but because the water 'has not *decided* to boil we do not need to refer to the consciousness of the water' (Bruce 1999: 12). However, any explanation of human society and human behaviour has to take into account the consciousness of the subject, because actions have meanings, which derive from consciousness. For these reasons the experimental method is impractical for sociologists.

This does not mean, however, that evidence need not be sought when sociologists generate and test theories. Despite apparent difficulties in establishing the 'truth', Bruce (1999: 17) argues, it is still possible to arrive at an accurate account of people's lives. He draws an analogy between sociological evidence and evidence in a court of law: in both cases, he suggests, it is possible to establish the truth from what appear to be contradictory accounts.

Question

Summarise the main differences between sociological methods of enquiry and those associated with the natural sciences.

The 'sociological imagination'

There is little doubt that sociology is one of the most controversial of all academic subjects, often giving rise to hostile reactions. Sociology has been associated with a radical and left-wing perspective, and despite the fact that sociologists such as Comte and Durkheim conceived of the subject in terms of describing and analysing what actually exists as opposed to speculating on what ought to exist, sociology has always been strongly associated with critiques of existing societies and speculation about the possibility of change. Zygmunt Bauman recognises that this questioning approach can invoke hostility: 'In an encounter with that familiar world ruled by habits … sociology acts as a meddlesome and often irritating stranger' (cited in Kirby et al. 1997: 3).

What critics might see as most questionable about the discipline of sociology, its practitioners see as its main strength. Anthony Giddens, for example, writes that the study of sociology is essentially liberating because 'it teaches appreciation of cultural variety and allows us an insight into the workings of social institutions' (cited in Kirby et al. 1997: 3). To 'do' sociology requires one to think in a specific way; fundamentally, it requires what C. Wright Mills describes as the *sociological imagination*. C. Wright Mills urges us to think outside our own experiences and look at what appears to us as

The concept of the **sociological imagination** refers to a specific way of thinking about the world, characterised by a willingness to think beyond our own experiences and to challenge commonsense or obvious explanations of human society and human behaviour.

'mundane' in a new light. Using the sociological imagination means departing from what are referred to as commonsense explanations: this implies an explanation of phenomena based on limited observations of human behaviour and our own, again limited, experiences of the social world. C. Wright Mills (1970) states that the sociological imagination enables three fundamental questions to be asked: (1) What is the structure of this particular society? (2) Where does this society stand in human history? (3) What varieties of men and women now prevail in this society and this period? What is important here is the questioning attitude to what is given, what is seen. Asking and answering all three questions ensures that no assumptions are made about what is being studied and that the context, both cultural and historical, is taken into account when considering any explanation of what is observed.

The **sociological imagination** is crucial to 'doing' sociology as it provides a critical and questioning edge, without which the discipline would be limited to simply describing social phenomena.

We seek to argue that without this critical and questioning edge, 'doing' sociology ceases to have any real purpose other than to describe, to provide background detail and a social context. Such an approach does not require one to ask the critical questions posed by C. Wright Mills, and neither, crucially, does it ask us to think about why social situations are as they are. One of the fundamental concerns of sociology is the distribution of power in society and its consequences. When, later in this book, you analyse inequalities in health you will see that social class is one of the main factors influencing levels of morbidity and mortality. What Chapter 6 will describe and analyse are not simply differences but inequalities in chances of good health and longevity. Inequality in terms of health is, literally, a matter of life and death. Social classes don't exist in isolation from one another, they form part of a social relationship; social disadvantage has another side and that is advantage. An understanding of theories of power is therefore essential to 'doing' sociology successfully.

Within the discipline of sociology, **theory** refers to attempts to provide systematic and consistent explanations of social phenomena. The term **paradigm** refers to a systematic way of thinking.

This chapter has drawn out what is unique about the discipline of sociology in terms of its subject matter, the nature of sociological evidence, methods of explanation and the mind-set described as the sociological imagination. The next section seeks to expand upon these themes by presenting an explanation of how sociologists explain social phenomena in terms of different theoretical perspectives.

1.2 An introduction to sociological theory

In this section we seek to explain and illustrate how sociologists explain the social world. To do this we will examine various competing theoretical approaches. To begin, however, it is necessary to think about what is meant by the term '**theory**' as a method of explanation. In commonsense terms a theory refers to a set of ideas or propositions used to explain and predict social phenomena. Our explanations derive ultimately from a particular perspective or worldview. Comte, for example, as we have already seen, divided human history into three phases, each characterised by a particular mode of thought (religious, metaphysical and scientific). Each of these modes of thought permits only certain kinds of explanation. The rational and scientific phase does not tolerate explanations that cannot be evidenced. Similarly, Seale and Pattison, in their study of the history of medicine, identify 'paradigms' or worldviews that characterised different stages in the development of medicine. Scientific medical knowledge is just one example of a medical **paradigm** (Seale and Pattison 1994: 28) and is based on what Seale and Pattison refer to as 'systematic investigation of all aspects of human biology … and includes experimental manipulation of body functions and testing of treatments under scientifically controlled conditions'.

Sociological theory and commonsense theory

Bruce argues that sociological explanations should share characteristics with scientific explanations in so far as they should be consistent, must accord with the evidence and must change if evidence can be found to refute them (Bruce 1999: 3). To the extent that this is true, it seems that sociological explanations differ from more commonsense explanations. It is possible to argue that the latter do not have to be supported by evidence and when evidence *is* produced there is little or no attempt to scrutinise its validity. Commonsense theories tend to be more in the nature of opinion than of fact. So far, then, this discussion has succeeded in establishing that sociological theory is characterised by the need to be consistent and evidenced. What also distinguishes sociological theory from commonsense theories is its ability to provide an 'account of the world which goes beyond what we can see and measure' (Marshall 1998: 666). 'Doing' and using sociological theory, therefore, enables us to explain phenomena of which we have no direct experience. Such a definition highlights what is unique and exciting about the discipline of sociology: its ability to inform us of differences and to think beyond our own experiences. Understanding the nature of sociological theory is a reminder of the importance of using the 'sociological imagination' as described by C. Wright Mills. Sociology is characterised by a range of different theoretical approaches, each providing a very different way of understanding social phenomena. The purpose of what follows is to provide you with an overview and introduction to these differing perspectives.

Doing and using sociological theory, enables us to explain phenomena of which we do not have direct experience.

Questions

What would be the main elements of a 'commonsense' theory about gender differences? How might this kind of explanation differ from a sociological explanation?

Functionalism

Functionalism offers an explanation of human society as a collection of inter-related substructures, the purpose of which is to sustain the overarching structure of society. As such, functionalism provides a 'consensual' representation of society, based on, first, an agreement to sustain society as it is and, second, on shared norms and beliefs.

The first approach to be examined is **functionalism**. This theoretical approach is based on an analogy between society and a biological organism. Just as the body is made up of different but interrelated and interdependent parts, so society is made up of a number of different systems and sub-systems. These different parts achieve unity in so far as they function to sustain the whole, in this example the wider social structure. Therefore, functionalism is less concerned with the individual and his or her aims, beliefs and consciousness, than with how our actions and beliefs function to maintain the system as a whole. An essential element in ensuring that the system is maintained is the cultural sub-system which ensures that individual motivations are in line with the values of the system as a whole. Without this central value system society would cease to function, because its cohesiveness could not be ensured. Each person has a certain role or function to fulfil, bounded by a certain set of expectations about how they will behave and how others should respond. These social expectations are referred to as role relationships, each of which carries with it a specific set of rights and obligations. The fulfilment of these roles and relationships ensures order and continuity in society.

Example

When a person takes on the 'sick role', they are excused from their normal roles and responsibilities. The medical profession determines who is legitimately 'sick'. This regulatory role ensures that not too many people are unable to fulfil their normal roles – otherwise illness would have a detrimental effect on the society as a whole.

In relation to the study of health and illness for example, the functionalist perspective is usefully illuminated by Talcott Parsons' concept of the 'sick role'. First, the concept is used to analyse sickness as a social role, not merely as a biological entity and physical experience. For any society to function smoothly, 'sickness' needs to be managed in such a way that the majority of people maintain their normal social roles and obligations. This perspective is based on the assumption that if too many people were to describe themselves as 'sick' and in need of being excused from their normal range of social obligations, this would be 'dysfunctional' in the sense of being disruptive for society as a whole. Those individuals who are judged by the medical profession as genuinely ill are only temporarily excused from normal obligations and then only if they comply with the rules of **the sick role**. Those people taking on the sick role do so only if they agree to comply with the regime given by the medical practitioner and if they are committed to getting well as soon as possible.

Links

Chapter 3, section 3.1 provides an illustration of the functionalist explanation of the doctor/patient relationship

The functionalist perspective is a consensual approach to understanding society, which also assumes that the latent or hidden functions of everyday activities have significance for maintaining the system as a whole. In relation to something as simple as eating, Lupton (1996) argues that the 'function' of food can be seen in broader terms than just as nutritional intake. A functionalist perspective serves to highlight the way in which 'food practices serve to support co-operative behaviour or structures of kinship in small groups' (Lupton 1996: 8). Lupton has also argued that the meal is a way of illustrating the culture of a specific society in terms of the order in which food is served (savoury then sweet) and the mixing of food types and temperatures.

However, the functionalist perspective has been subject to much criticism. In relation to the sick role, for example, it has been suggested that Parsons overlooked the potential for conflict between the patient and the practitioner and that he misguidedly assumed that the practitioner would always act in the best interests of the patient. However, the main criticism is that it is an unproven assumption that situations have a fixed, obvious and shared meaning.

Symbolic interactionism

In contrast, **symbolic interactionism** is based on the premise that there is a fundamental difference between the subject matter of sociology and that of the natural sciences. While the study of the natural world deals with physical, inanimate objects, the subject matter of sociology consists of people whose actions are motivated by human consciousness. Symbolic interactionism is, therefore, concerned with how people see and understand the social world. This theoretical approach is concerned less with the larger social system or structure than with interpreting human behaviour. As with the 'sociological imagination', the emphasis here is on looking again at the most common sense and commonplace aspects of our culture and questioning what we assume to be 'natural' and 'normal'.

The significance of this approach can be seen in relation to understanding health behaviour that appears to be irrational. Graham (1993) examined patterns of cigarette smoking among mothers on low incomes. What is revealed is

Symbolic interactionism explains social phenomena from the perspective of its participants. An essential element of this theoretical perspective is the unique nature of the social world as made up of the actions of participants motivated by human consciousness. The meaning of human action cannot, therefore, be observed or assumed, but must be interpreted by studying the meanings that people attach to their behaviour.

In the context of this discussion, **micro** refers to the small-scale aspects of human behaviour, for example why individuals embark on criminal activities. **Macro** refers to the larger, structural aspects of society. In terms of criminal activities, this might involve an analysis of the economic circumstances of criminals, an analysis of law making and law enforcement, as well as of the role of the state in regulating such behaviour.

relatively high levels of spending on cigarettes in low-income households. In terms of what can be observed or assumed, this behaviour might well indicate a degree of irrationality in that it contradicts dominant health messages about the dangers of smoking, and diverts limited financial resources from the family. Graham, however, favours a theoretical approach dependent upon the symbolic interactionism tradition of interpreting human behaviour in the context of people's own beliefs and meanings. This alternative interpretation associates cigarette smoking with the maintenance of normal, caring routines in that smoking creates a 'space' between the mothers and their children, providing 'time out' from the demanding routines of caring. 'Viewed within the context of mothers' daily lives, cigarette smoking appears to be a way of coping with the constant and unremitting demands of caring: a way of temporarily escaping without leaving the room' (Graham 1993: 93).

What the interactionist tradition presents us with is insight into two important aspects of social phenomena: first, in terms of the emphasis placed on the disputed nature of meaning we are clearly reminded of what is central to the discipline itself, namely the questioning of the taken-for-granted. Second, the focus is on what are referred to as the **micro** elements of society, that is, the small-scale interactions between individuals and between individuals and groups. An overview of the research based on this approach indicates both the strengths and weaknesses of symbolic interactionism. Becker's (1974) analysis of deviance is an excellent illustration of the symbolic interactionist perspective. The definition of deviance that Becker offers does not assume that what is described as deviant is fixed for all time, or that different cultures have the same definition of what counts as deviant. Becker's analysis focuses instead on the understanding of the meaning of deviance and the way in which that definition may be considered fluid rather than static. Becker defines deviance as any act that is perceived as such. Deviance is a label attached to the behaviour of an individual, rather than a quality of their behaviour. His own research tended to concentrate on certain types of 'deviant' behaviour such as illicit drug use and prostitution, the process that led to an individual taking on a deviant career, the factors that sustained him or her in that deviant career, and the processes whereby deviant behaviour became labelled as such. Becker's research concentrated less on the structural factors that might help explain crime and deviance, such as poverty and placed little emphasis on the source of power of those agencies, such as criminal justice agencies, who label some people deviant. Becker talked of 'moral entrepreneurs' as influential shapers of public morals but made little or no attempt to place these individuals and groups within the social context of society. In other words, the **macro** elements of the social structure were given much less emphasis.

Marxism

Strictly speaking Marx did not set out to be a sociologist and it was mainly with the political radicalisation of the 1960s that his ideas became part of the sociological mainstream. His ideas, however, do provide powerful insights into the structure of society, suggesting that it is the economic structure of any society that determines the social relations contained within that structure. It is the distribution of the ownership of the means of production that gives rise to specific patterns of class relations, which, crucially, in all societies are characterised by inequalities of power. Marx described modern societies in the west as capitalist, that is to say divided between those who privately own the means of production (a minority) and those who are dependent on selling their labour power to make a living (the majority). This classic division provides a description of the two main classes, the bourgeoisie and the proletariat. The relationship between the two is unequal, primarily in that the relations of production result in the exploitation of the latter in a way that is systematic and oppressive.

Marxist theory is used to question the 'naturalness' of capitalist relations and to unmask the reality of what is fundamentally an exploitative relationship. This theoretical approach is representative of the structural analysis of society, less concerned with the 'micro' elements and more concerned with the larger picture, the underlying factors that explain social, economic and political relationships. Marxist theory, therefore, is a distinct sociological perspective, a tool for our analysis of the social structure. It would be a mistake to assume that all that this theoretical perspective can offer us is an appreciation of the significance of economic factors on, for example, health chances. Such an approach would lose sight of what Marxist theory can provide us with in terms of a critique of existing social, economic and political relationships. Vicente Navarro's analysis (Moon and Gillespie 1995: 73) of the causes of ill health and the relationship between the state and the medical profession is based on such insights. What Navarro provides us with is an explanation both of the causes of inequalities of health between different social classes and of why this situation continues and is, as he argues, maintained by the medical profession.

The key to this situation is, Navarro suggests, to be found in the alliance of interests between the ruling classes and the medical profession; each, for different reasons, derives power from the continuation of these conditions of inequality. For the ruling classes, health inequalities are an indication of the difference in life chances that exist between themselves and the working classes in particular. The provision of health care through a system such as the National Health Service is largely about maintaining a reasonable level of health among the working classes,

Marxism explains social phenomena as primarily determined by the economic structure of society. Social change, it is argued, is the product of changes in economic relationships. In the context of the modern period the advent of capitalism and industrialisation produced social divisions based on the ownership or non-ownership of property. The economic inequalities that result from ownership or non-ownership of property are the starting point for understanding why there are inequalities in health between the middle and the working classes.

sufficient to ensure that people are able to work and be returned to work following illness. Navarro in part explains the medical profession's alliance with the ruling classes in terms of their shared willingness to perpetuate the belief that the principal causes of ill health are personal and physical rather than social. Such a situation in turn strengthens the position of the medical profession in explaining illness to the lay population but also, significantly, fosters a dependency on medicine to cure illness and disease. To admit that patterns of disease and illness are largely determined by economic and social factors would be to rob the medical profession of ideological dominance, which is founded on the claim that it is medical advances and medical technology that have produced the most startling improvements in the health of the nation. Therefore, the alliance between the ruling classes and the medical profession serves the interests of both by maintaining the professional dominance of the latter and by sustaining a reasonably healthy working population for the former.

Feminism

Feminism is a broad concept that explains social structures as fundamentally based on inequalities between women and men. In general, feminist sociologists have challenged the traditional preoccupation of the discipline with the effects of industrialisation and the world of paid work and institutional politics. Such an approach, it is argued, has ignored significant elements of society such as the family and gender relationships.

Marxist theory has been criticised in particular for its almost exclusive emphasis on the economic determinants of social relationships and for the resulting primacy of social class in any analysis of inequality. *Feminist theory* from the 1960s onwards sought to challenge what was seen as the invisibility of gender in sociological theory. Giddens suggests that sociology has as its main focus 'the study of the social institutions brought into being by the industrial transformations of the past two or three centuries' (Giddens 1997: 8). Feminist critics argued that the founding fathers of sociology were concerned with a narrow range of topics such as social class, the division of labour in industrial society and the role of the state.

It is possible to argue that two essential elements of this social transformation were largely overlooked. The first relates to the way in which industrialisation impacted specifically upon women, compared to men. According to Ramazanaglu (1989) one of the most significant changes for women related to the shift of work for remuneration from the home (or near the home) to a separate and distinct space, such as the factory. Such a split set up for the first time the dilemma of how to combine 'work' and childcare. The second element illuminates the practical changes in women's lives as well as conceptual shifts in explanations of social phenomena. The modern era is associated with a perceived split between the 'public' and the 'private' spheres. It was assumed that the natural area of study for sociology was the 'public' world of paid work, politics and the state. Since these were also the areas where men were dominant, it was this aspect of the social world that came to be associated with them. Women, on the other hand, remained within the 'private' sphere of the home, family and unpaid work. The former sphere was clearly seen as open to change, while the latter was assumed to be unchanging and 'natural'. The result of this conceptual split was an unquestioning acceptance of women and men as fundamentally different from one another and an assumption that these 'natural' differences could not be altered.

Links

Chapter 4 includes a discussion of the male dominance of medicine in relation to reproductive technology.

As a challenge to these assumptions, feminist theory can make a substantial contribution to our understanding of the social world in general and to the study of health and illness in particular. Feminist theory provides, for example, an analysis of gender relations on the basis of the way in which female inequality has been structured and maintained in society. One rather controversial concept used to explain this inequality is that of **patriarchy**, literally meaning the rule of men over women and of older men over younger men. In terms of uncovering what is distinct about women's lives as compared to men's, the concept of patriarchy provides a unique insight into many aspects of women's lives. Writers such as Oakley (1984) have argued that women's lives have been subject to far greater control and regulation by the medical profession than have men's. Particular examples can be seen in relation to pregnancy and childbirth, where what was previously seen as a 'natural' event attended by women rapidly became the focus of medical intervention, and now principally takes place in hospital, with the profession of obstetrics being dominated by men.

Postmodernism

The final theoretical approach to be discussed in this chapter is less a school of thought than part of a recent critical and challenging questioning of traditional sociological theory. Postmodernism refers to the present historical period characterised by the globalisation of the economy and culture, and by a fragmentation of individual identity such that old certainties of class, national and gender identity are called into question. The term 'postmodern' also refers to a particular paradigm or worldview. In this case, what is being challenged is the certainty of our knowledge about the world, the ability of sociological theory to uncover the 'truth' about the social

Postmodernist theories veer away from all-embracing theories such as those described above that attempt to explain all social phenomena. Instead, the emphasis is on the impossibility of uncovering the 'truth' about society. Postmodernism draws our attention to how our knowledge of the social world is constructed, and offers a critical and questioning approach to understanding the world around us.

Medical knowledge is an example of an established body of thought that is challenged by postmodernism as just one interpretation of reality. In other words, the 'truth' of medical knowledge is challenged.

Discourse refers to a specific way of thinking about and conceptualising a particular subject. The essence of a discourse is the language used to express thoughts. Science is an example of a discourse that rules out some kinds of explanations (for example spiritual) and only allows for others (for example, rational and evidenced 'facts').

world, and the desirability of this. Thus, the emphasis of this particular approach is less on producing an all-embracing theory which explains all aspects of the social structure, and more on enquiring into the nature of knowledge itself.

Michel Foucault argued that in order to understand science and medicine we have to think about them as 'discourses' about the body, health and the natural world, rather than accepting these disciplines as objective descriptions of reality. The concept of **discourse** is an important one within contemporary sociology and represents a distinct way of thinking, seeing and conversing about particular phenomena, all of which create a virtual 'arena', ruling some ways of thinking as legitimate and others as not. Medicine is often described as a dominant *discourse* in relation to the study of health, disease and the body because western biomedicine has become the accepted, and therefore legitimate, way of thinking, talking about and seeing these aspects of human experience. Medicine represents one discourse on health, disease and the body and Foucault draws our attention to previous, non-scientific explanations of disease and perceptions of the body. Post-modernist theory makes two main contributions to the study of health and disease: first, we are offered a way of challenging the dominance of medicine and questioning what appears to be scientific, true and objective. Second, we can appreciate the way in which knowledge discourses can be used to discipline us. According to Bilton et al. (1996), medicine cannot be seen, then, as merely and actively associated with clinical healing; 'the medicalisation of the body … has to be understood as a process of social control' (Bilton et al. 1996: 424). We have seen from the earlier example of feminist theory and the critique of the regulation of pregnancy and childbirth that the application of medical techniques and knowledge often results in the control and regulation of patients.

Conclusion

This chapter has sought to establish the nature of the discipline of sociology by detailing what is distinctive about its subject matter and method of enquiry. You have also been introduced to various theoretical explanations of social phenomena. Only by having such theoretical perspectives are we able to glimpse what is beneath the commonsense surface perceptions. In the rest of the book you will see how this distinctive way of looking at the world helps to bring about an understanding of health in its fullest and widest sense. What will emerge is that health is clearly bound up with the social world, with some of the main inequalities and patterns of health and illness only explainable by reference to sociology.

SUMMARY POINTS

- Sociology is concerned with the study of society and specifically with key issues such as inequalities in life chances.
- Sociology offers what Bruce (1999) terms a 'scientific' method of enquiry characterised by the search for valid evidence.
- The study of sociology requires us to think outside our own experiences and to employ the 'sociological imagination'.
- Sociological theory can be distinguished from 'everyday theory' by its requirement to resort to reasoned, evidenced and coherent explanations of social phenomena.

Taking your studies further

This chapter will have helped you understand many of the key terms, concepts, theories and debates relating to sociological theory. Listed below are journal articles and books that will provide deeper and more detailed discussions of the points raised in this chapter. You will also find what is available on the companion website. This offers downloads of relevant material, plus links to useful websites in addition to podcasts and other features.

Recommended reading

Benton, T. and Craib, I. (2001) *Philosophy of Social Science: The Philosophical Foundations of Social Thought*. Basingstoke: Palgrave.

Bruce, S. (1999) *Sociology: A Very Short Introduction*. Oxford: Oxford University Press.

Craib, I. (2004) *Classical Social Theory: An Introduction to the Thought of Marx, Weber, Durkheim and Simmel*. Oxford: Oxford University Press.

Scambler, G. (2002) *Health and Social Change: A Critical Theory*. Buckingham: Open University Press.

On the companion website

Scott, J.P. (2004) *Social Theory: Central Issues in Sociology*. London: Sage. Chapter 1.

2

Concepts of health and medicine

MAIN POINTS

- Modern medicine emerges out of the Enlightenment, a critical historical period when society became secular and scientific: this replaced religious explanations of the natural world.
- The medical model of health stresses a mechanistic view of the body and a reliance on biological causation to explain illness.
- The social model provides a holistic approach stressing that health and illness can only be explained by analysing the social.
- Foucault's concept of the clinical gaze draws our attention to how medicine observes and treats the body as a physical entity devoid of reference to the person.

KEY CONCEPTS

The Enlightenment, science, rationality, paradigm, social model, medical model, bedside medicine, clinical medicine, laboratory medicine, and the clinical gaze.

Introduction

The aims of this chapter are twofold: to provide a historical account of the development of modern medicine and to examine the social construction of medical knowledge. We employ the concept of the **sociological imagination** to stress the necessity of a historical and questioning approach to the study of medicine and the development of the medical profession.

Medicine represents a specific type of knowledge about the human body that is applied to either care for or cure of the recipient of medical treatment. In order to understand the practice of medicine at the present time, it is necessary to know how it developed historically. This chapter seeks to explain two main elements of medical knowledge: first, its historical origins and, second, the type of knowledge underpinning the practice of medicine.

The Enlightenment refers to a body of thought, first developed in the eighteenth century, which challenged explanations of the world based on religious or superstitious explanations. Enlightenment thought, on the other hand, was based on a commitment to rational, secular and scientific explanations.

2.1 The development of modern medicine: science, rationality and the legacy of the Enlightenment

Before we begin to examine medical perspectives on the body, it would be helpful to ascertain the origins of these ideas. According to Stacey (1988) various cultural, social and economic factors, all of which have their origins in the eighteenth-century Enlightenment, help explain the development of modern medicine. The term **the Enlightenment** refers to a body of thought rather than to a specific period in European history. Underpinning this intellectual movement was a strong emphasis on reason rather than belief, superstition or even religious thought. The Enlightenment is traditionally associated with rationality and the search for evidence. It was anticipated that on the basis of rational, reasoned and evidenced thought traditional institutions and ideas could be replaced with 'modern' practices. This element of the Enlightenment paved the way for a secular understanding of **society** and of people's place within it. The application of reason to human life, it was argued, opened up the possibility of the advancement of the human race by uncovering the massive potential of *science* and reason. Stacey (1988: 47) argues that the developments that took place laid the basis from which biomedicine developed, led to its domination over all alternative healing systems and established a division of health labour that its practitioners also dominated.

In the first instance, the growing **secularisation** of society opened the way for alternative, scientific explanations for disease. 'Medical' labels and 'scientific' explanations could be used to understand the origins of disease and their potential cures. Chapter 9,

The concept of **science** is associated with the study of the natural and physical world, characterised by observation, measurement, experimentation and objectivity. **Secularisation** refers to the acceptance of non-religious explanations of the world.

which examines mental health, will illustrate these arguments in detail. Explanations of 'madness' in spiritual terms or in terms of 'possession' gave way to explanations drawn from the examination of the body and brain based on empirical observation and the recording of the underlying physical, organic cause. This drive to uncover the specific aetiology of a disease by examining the human body is exemplified in the desire to explore the bodies of the dead as well as the living. The search for knowledge about the body encouraged early medical practitioners to act unlawfully by taking possession of cadavers procured illicitly. This illegal trade thrived despite the fact that practitioners already enjoyed access to the bodies of the poor and destitute who had died in workhouses and other institutions.

Questions

How important for the medical profession is the continuing use of bodies for research and teaching? What is the connection between the decline in religious belief and the greater use of bodies for research and teaching?

Edinburgh was notorious for its 'body snatchers' or 'resurrectionists', principally because of its strong tradition of medical education. The best known practitioners of this trade were Burke and Hare who, in the early part of the nineteenth century, also murdered to provide corpses. When captured, the latter turned king's evidence, while Burke was hanged in front of a crowd of 20,000 and his own body later dissected in the same way as those he had procured. A wallet made from Burke's skin can still be seen within the Medical School at Edinburgh University.

Visitors to older Edinburgh graveyards must have noticed their strange resemblance to zoological gardens, the rows of iron cages suggesting rather the dens of wild animals than the quiet resting places of the dead. And, in fact, these barred and grated cells were designed as a protection against human wolves who nightly prowled about such places in quest of prey, and furnish very real testimony to the fears by which our forebears were beset respecting the security of the sepulchres ... . It is obvious that the lawful supply of subjects was wholly inadequate to meet the growing needs of the new [medical] school ... the surgeons and barbers' apprentices had been in use diligently to till the soil and reap the harvest of what had been finely called 'Death's mailing'. ... At first zealous apprentices were the only body snatchers, but owing to the popularity of the Edinburgh medical school and the great increase of students, there arose a class of men who, adopting as a business the raising of the dead, became known as the Resurrectionists. (Roughhead 1921: 152)

The Enlightenment underpinned the development of specific *methods* of investigation in relation to medicine, namely scientific methods. The superiority of scientific thought was said to lie in the fact that evidence and theories were derived not from belief but from observation, and were confirmed through a process of experimentation. Evidence developed in this way was seen as unbiased, *rational* and purely descriptive of the natural world. Scientific facts could not be disputed except by employing the same methods to question or disprove an assertion. In Chapter 4 we will examine **alternative medicine** and see that the same assumed superiority of scientific methods is still used to question the validity of practices such as homoeopathy.

> Science's ability to provide rational explanations continues to be one of its main strengths. **Rational** means adherence to a logical and tenable process of explanation.

2.2 Medical perspectives on the body, health and illness

Biomedicine is the principal way of understanding health and illness in western culture, being widely accepted not just by the medical profession but also by the lay (non-professional) population. There is general agreement among contributors to debates in medical sociology that the *medical model* of explanation has a number of defining characteristics. Nettleton, for example, describes five features (Nettleton 1995: 5).

> The **medical model** is a specific way of thinking about and explaining disease based on biological factors.

1 *Mind–body dualism.* This refers to an acceptance that when treating disease the mind and the body can be treated as two separate entities. The physical body rather than the more problematic 'mind' is *the* subject of medicine. Medicine's appropriation of the body is such that, until recently, there was very little written by sociologists about the body; this was the domain of the medical profession.
2 *Mechanical metaphor.* Nettleton uses this concept to draw our attention to the way in which medicine is said to view the body as a machine, the functioning of which is determined by biological and scientific laws. Having knowledge of how the body functions allows medical practitioners to 'repair' any dysfunction.
3 *Technological imperative.* This refers to the significance attached to medical methods of intervention, whether pharmacological or surgical, in treating the body. As we shall see, there is often a tendency to overemphasise the curative element of biomedicine and underplay the beneficial contributions made by, for example, changes in diet or environment. While the development of medical technology brings with it considerable benefits, these developments also have a cost, for instance in terms of the harmful consequences either of medicines or of medical intervention.
4 Biomedicine is described by Nettleton as 'reductionist' in that there is a tendency to reduce all explanations to the physical workings of the body. There is an echo of this *reductionist tendency* in the dualistic nature of medicine as well as in the significance attached to the 'technological imperative' in the primary

role attached to all things physical. One of the major criticisms of the medical model stems from its apparent unwillingness to acknowledge that both social and psychological factors influence health.

5   The *doctrine of specific aetiology* refers to the belief that all disease originates from specific and knowable causes.

Such a description of the medical model may well strike you as rather rigid, and as a far more accurate account of medicine and medical practice in the past rather than today. We would argue, however, that central elements of medical knowledge remain but that medicine is a dynamic body of thought, capable of changing and adapting in the light of new discoveries. The fluid nature of medical knowledge means that some elements of the medical model may be more or less important now than they were in the past.

Links

A more detailed discussion of the body and chronic illness is provided in Chapter 10

It is perhaps easier to see the relevance of such a model in the past, when infectious diseases were the main cause of morbidity and mortality. The major killers of the twentieth and twenty-first centuries are long-term, chronic illnesses. What distinguishes these conditions from diseases of the past is that their causes are 'social'. Heart disease is the main cause of death in Scotland and some cities like Glasgow, for example, have particularly high rates. While some causes of heart disease can be traced back to a specific dysfunction of the organ, the principal cause is an unhealthy lifestyle. It may be difficult to defend the medical model as outlined by Nettleton when public awareness campaigns attach such a degree of significance to individuals changing their lifestyles rather than to the medical profession repairing what appears simply to be a faulty machine. Pharmaceuticals such as lipids may be able to reduce the harmful effects of heart disease and hypertension but they cannot eradicate the disease.

Authors such as Lupton (1995) have urged us to consider the way in which the medical model has developed and reinvented itself to the point where it can embrace social as well as psychological factors. It is, therefore, not always appropriate to contrast the medical model of medicine with the *social model* of medicine. The social dimensions of heart disease is a topical example of this, as is the recent acknowledgement by the British Medical Association that diseases such as ME have both a physical and a psychological dimension. It would be a mistake to accept the medical model as a static representation of medical thought and practice. Medicine and medical practice are no longer solely concerned with the biological and the physical but, because of the changing nature of disease, are able to place disease and the diseased body in a social context. Medicine goes beyond simply treating disease and is now actively engaged in a moral crusade to change the way in which people live, and to influence the choices that they make. Turner (1994) suggests that the growth in the influence of medicine over our lives, coupled with the demise of religious influence, has resulted in a new moral order: 'the doctor has replaced the priest as the custodian of social values' (1994: 37). This 'moralistic' element of medicine cannot be adequately accounted for in terms of the five characteristics identified above. In order to embrace the modern dimensions of medicine and medical practice we have to be prepared to extend the traditional medical model to a more complex body of thought that can and does embrace social and psychological aspects of health and disease.

2.3 'Medical paradigms': the social construction of medical knowledge

Thus far, this chapter has explored the intellectual and cultural origins of medicine and provided an account of the main characteristics of the medical model. The significance of this discussion, and that of other chapters that follow, is that it allows the student of **sociology** to place the development of medicine within a historical context, and thus fulfils one of the essential criteria of the request to employ the 'sociological imagination'. The second objective of this chapter is to explain the social construction of medical knowledge.

Social constructionism is characterised by an emphasis on the extent to which 'society' is actively and creatively produced by human beings. The world is portrayed as made or invented – rather than as given or taken for granted. 'Social worlds are interpretive nets woven by individuals and groups' (Marshall 1998: 609). The extent to which medical knowledge can also be said to be socially constructed, that is, the degree to which medical knowledge is a product of those engaged in its practice, can be illustrated by Jewson's concept of *paradigms* of medical knowledge. The term **paradigm** refers to a model or mode of thought, a particular way of seeing the world, that sets boundaries to *what* we see, *how* we might measure and record that information and *which* factors are significant and which are not.

Paradigms of knowledge shift and change over time, as illustrated by the earlier discussion of the medical model, and, therefore, offer us a way of conceptualising the fluid and dynamic nature of medical knowledge.

Bedside medicine	Clinical medicine	Laboratory medicine
• disease as a total 'Psychosomatic' experience • lay and 'medical' practitioners • place of treatment: home	• specific aetiology of diseases • specialist practitioners in possession of specialist knowledge about the body • Place of treatment: hospital	• disease as a 'biochemical disturbance' • specialist practitioners, knowledge of cellular construction of the body • Place of treatment: laboratory

FIGURE 2.1   *Jewson's three paradigms of medical knowledge (Seale and Pattison 1994)*

Figure 2.1 represents a simplification of the three paradigms. It is a useful starting point in the **analysis** of the social construction of medical knowledge and raises the following significant points:

- Medical knowledge has changed and developed over time. What was once held as a reasonable explanation may later be disputed and cast aside. Early medical theories of hysteria, for example, maintained that the womb of 'hysterical' women moved around the body.
- Medical knowledge and, more generally, knowledge about health and disease has become increasingly specialised, focusing first on the 'whole' person, then on specific parts of the body and finally, analysing the construction of cells. Theoretical knowledge of the body, learned knowledge, has taken precedence over experiential knowledge. Medicine and medical practice has increasingly become the preserve of those educated and trained by current practitioners and registered with their professional bodies. Lay practitioners, such as lay midwives, were systematically excluded from the practice of medicine.
- Each paradigm shift in thought has entailed a shift in the nature of the relationship between the practitioner and the patient. The 'bedside manner' paradigm suggests that, at least in the case of the wealthy, practitioners were 'patronised' by clients. Clients paid directly for the service and those providing it were often considered their social inferiors; power lay with the patient. If you compare and contrast this with the quality of, and the balance of power in, the contemporary relationship between practitioner and patient, a very different picture emerges. Despite the clear benefits which derive from the provision of a National Health Service, the position of general practitioners as 'independent contractors' within the service means that payment is not gained directly from the patient but via the Health Service itself. It could be argued that because of this the service provided is organised around the needs of the practitioners rather than of the patients. Appointment times might be one example. Most appointments are offered within the confines of the working day and, with the exception of emergencies, only on Monday to Friday. Given this, for many people in work it is hard to find a suitable time to see a GP without taking time off paid work.

The paradigm that accords best with our experiences of medicine in contemporary terms is that of clinical or hospital medicine. The following discussion provides a more detailed consideration of this aspect of medical knowledge and practice.

2.4 Foucault and the clinical gaze

The concept of the **clinical gaze** is associated with Foucault and refers to a specific way of conceptualising the body, rather than simply describing the physical location of the examination. This new conceptualisation of the body stemmed from a number of developments, some of which have been mentioned in the discussion above. For example, the Enlightenment gave rise to the dominance of scientific and rational thought, an essential element of which was the opportunity to see the physical body as part of the 'natural' world. Part of this way of conceptualising the body is based on the idea of the mind/body split, enabling us to perceive the body as a physical object outside, external and separate to us as represented by the mind.

The concept of the **clinical gaze** is part of a specific discourse on the body in which the body is perceived as a physical object capable of being observed, measured and treated with little or no reference to the person.

Links

Chapter 10, section 10.2 explains the central role of medicine in interpreting the human body.

The contested nature of knowledge is explored in Chapter 1, section 1.3 in a general discussion of postmodernism.

The ability to conceive of the body as an object in part stemmed from the increasing trend towards its physical dissection. The corpse became the source of knowledge about the body and that knowledge was the domain of medical science. The concept of the clinical gaze was used by Foucault (1973) to describe a specific and distinct method of examination and understanding, made possible by the physical examination of the internal workings of the body. Foucault's analysis contains the possibility of extending our knowledge of the socially constructed nature of reality. What may appear to us as real – for example, the physical make-up of the body – is actually the outcome of a specific kind of knowledge. To interpret the body and its workings requires a 'guide' because the body and its functions are not self-evident. Our representations of the body, whether through models or through diagrams, are the product of how we understand it. Without some training in what to look for and some general acceptance of the functions of the different parts of the anatomy, it is argued, we would not be able to interpret what we see. A map of a geographical area is a representation of it, full of complex signs and symbols that help us interpret what we see. The map is not an accurate representation of what we actually see as we walk about a city, but it is a guide that helps us interpret what we see. In the same way, medical knowledge provides a guide by which to read the body.

That medical science does not represent 'reality' can be illustrated with reference to explanations once held as 'true' but since revised in the light of new knowledge. The example of medical understanding of the blood is a useful illustration. As late as 1750 the nature and function of blood was interpreted in a very different way from today. It is worth remembering that this belief dominated despite the discovery of the circulation of the blood by the English physician William Harvey in 1628.

Working with the understanding that there are two independent systems of blood vessels, the arteries and the veins, Galen [Greek physician, second century AD] believed that some almost immaterial vivifying substance (that is to say a substance endowing life), *pneuma*, was brought in from the air when we breathe, taken to the lungs and from there to the left chamber of the heart, where it was mixed with ordinary blood and was then drawn into the arteries. Its life possessing and life giving properties were evident to the senses when it was compared with the blood in the veins; arterial blood was bright, frothy, it spurted when the artery was cut, it needed the strong walls of the arteries to contain its natural tendency to expansion, and it had the pulse of life. Venous blood, by contrast was slow moving, and the thinner walls of its vessels showed no pulse. (Cunningham 1994: 62)

The physical examination of the body provided the opportunity to distinguish between normal and abnormal functions. On this basis, it is hardly surprising that the dominant definition of 'health' is as the absence of disease, and that medicine is so closely associated with the treatment of dysfunction rather than the promotion of health. The physical setting of the clinic or the hospital provided practitioners with the opportunity to examine bodies in large numbers and establish concepts of normality and abnormality. The benefits of such a distinction are clear. Practitioners are able to distinguish between a working kidney and one that is malfunctioning. We know that it is normal for babies to be born with a fontanelle, but in cases where this gap has prematurely closed surgery is necessary to allow the brain to develop normally. The question of normality and abnormality seems unproblematic in cases such as these. Sociologists of health and illness are concerned, however, that such judgements extend further to embrace human behaviour and lifestyles, for example in relation to mental health and well-being. What begins to emerge from this analysis is a picture of medicine and medical practice as both caring and potentially controlling, suggesting as it does what is normal and abnormal. The next chapter examines these issues in detail.

This chapter has explored the development of modern medicine by providing a historical account of the belief systems that gave rise to the practices that are still with us today.

Conclusion

Medicine as a distinct scientific body of knowledge did not just come into being by 'itself' or by chance. Certain social and historical circumstances were necessary for its development. This occurred in the eighteenth century during the Enlightenment, a period when religious explanations and understandings of the natural world gave way to secular and scientific understandings. At this point it became increasingly legitimate to seek explanations of disease and illness with reference to the biological workings of the body as opposed to explanations which made reference to divine sanctions or superstitious causes.

This initial focus on the body shaped the future development of medicine. Biological systems, and particularly their failures, became the dominant perspective of medicine over more holistic accounts of the causes and cures of illness. This has seen medicine favouring a mechanical metaphor of the body, with technology and science as being the best (if not the only) ways to treat illness. As the rest of this book discusses, health and illness cannot be explained solely by reference to the internal workings of the biological body. What happens with the body is only one aspect of the whole 'story' of health.

SUMMARY POINTS

- This chapter has explained the development of modern medicine as a specific form of knowledge about the human body.
- The development of medical knowledge is strongly associated with science, rationality and the Enlightenment.
- Scientific medical knowledge represents a specific way of seeing and understanding the functions of the body. One example of this is the traditional idea of the mind/body split.
- Medical knowledge is dynamic and evolving.
- The possession of specialist medical knowledge leads to an increasing tendency to engage with the disease rather than with the patient.
- Medical knowledge is a form of power, with the potential to control and influence the lives of its recipients.

Case study

Imagine that you are being asked to publicly debate the use of embryos in medical research. Embryonic materials can be used to grow stem cells that in turn can be used to develop replacement organs for those that have failed and thus, ultimately, to save and prolong human lives. You are encountering strong resistance from the opposing side, made up of religious groups who oppose the use of embryos in medical research.

1   On what grounds might religious groups protest about the use of embryos to grow stem cells?
2   What arguments could you produce to allow this kind of research to continue?
3   On a personal level, reflect upon your own feelings about this kind of research.

Taking your studies further

This chapter will have helped you understand many of the key terms, concepts, theories and debates relating to health and medicine. Listed below are journal articles and books that will provide deeper and more detailed discussions of the points raised in this chapter. You will also find what is available on the companion website. This offers downloads of relevant material, plus links to useful websites in addition to podcasts and other features.

Recommended reading

Books

Foucault, M. (1973) *The Birth of the Clinic: An Archaeology of Medical Perception*. London: Random House.

Lupton, D. (2003) *Medicine as Culture: Illness, Disease and the Body in Western Societies*, 2nd edn. London: SAGE.

Stacey, M. (1988) *The Sociology of Health and Healing*. London: Routledge.

Journals

Calnan, M., Wainwright, D., O'Neill, C., Winterbottom, A. and Watkins, C. (2007) 'Illness action rediscovered: a case study of upper limb pain', *Sociology of Health and Illness*, 29 (3): 321–46.

On the companion website

Tausing, M., Subedi, S. and Subedi, J. (2007) 'The bioethics of medical research in very poor countries', *Health*, 11 (4): 145–61.

3

Medical power and knowledge

MAIN POINTS

- The medical profession exerts a great deal of power in society, though current social policy developments seek to limit clinical autonomy.
- Some medical decisions can create and lead to illness.
- Public health measures can lead to surveillance and control of people's lives beyond their health.

KEY CONCEPTS

Power, clinical autonomy, the clinical method, surveillance.

Introduction

The purpose of this chapter is to consider the implications of the **power** of the medical profession. The nature and extent of this power can be understood in a positive sense (caring for) in terms of improving our quality of life and extending our span of life. However, a sociological **analysis** of medical power must take cognisance of the way in which this same ability can also be used as a means of controlling and regulating human lives. Like Bob the Builder, the medical profession, in most cases, can answer the question 'Can we fix it?' with an emphatic 'Yes we can!' The power of medicine is beyond doubt, but simply saying we can do something does not imply that we should. To say, for example, we can clone animals is not the same thing as saying that we should. Developments within modern medicine have meant that what in the past may have been purely clinical decisions are now ethical decisions. For example, the age at which premature babies can survive has steadily decreased, raising the question of at what stage of pregnancy terminations should be permitted. Medical staff have increasingly found themselves trying, on the one hand, to maintain the life of one child and on the other, aborting a foetus of the same age.

The meaning of the concept of **power** is the subject of much debate within sociology. In the context of this discussion, however, the concept refers to (a) the ability to ensure that a particular point of view prevails in a disputed situation, (b) the capacity to ensure that someone acts in a certain way, and (c) the ability to stifle opposition to a particular perspective.

3.1 'Clinical autonomy': Doctor knows best

The concept of **clinical autonomy** is best understood as the freedom of clinicians to make decisions on the basis of their professional judgement and specialist knowledge. Doctors are not unique in claiming this level of autonomy; most professions make similar claims on the basis of the possession of an exclusive body of knowledge and a specialist education. Doctors, dentists, lawyers, nurses and even dieticians have their claim to specialist knowledge and judgement supported by the state in the form of state registration. Only those who have fulfilled the necessary training and experience are allowed to practise.

Clinical autonomy therefore suggests freedom to both diagnose and treat patients with appropriate means. As Seale and Pattison (1994: 100) comment, the **clinical method** itself is premised on 'an overriding orientation towards action'. (see Figure 3.1)

Challenges to this degree of clinical freedom have come from a variety of sources. Patients are generally better informed about their condition than in the past, and those with chronic long-term conditions can accumulate an impressive level of knowledge and understanding of their illness. Cultural and political developments

The concept of **clinical autonomy** refers to the freedom of clinicians to make decisions on the basis of their professional judgement and specialist knowledge. This definition implies the downgrading of other assessments of the same situation.

Diagnosis – take a history – define symptoms – examination – signs – prognosis

FIGURE 3.1   *The clinical method (Seale and Pattison 1994)*

have encouraged us to see ourselves as consumers of health care, with resulting rights to adequate treatment and recourse if we feel that the treatment has not been appropriate. A second challenge has come from alternative practitioners who have raised serious questions about the effectiveness of conventional treatments and their potentially damaging long-term effects.

Health managers' attempts to curb the power of clinicians

A third challenge to clinical autonomy has come from within the National Health Service itself in terms of various reforms that have sought to enhance the power of managers to control the activities of clinicians. Proposals made in the 1989 White Paper *Working for Patients*, and later enacted in the 1990 NHS and Community Care Act, aimed at curtailing the power of clinicians. Any attempt to control and regulate expenditure in the NHS, it was argued, must encompass the activities of clinicians. Decisions made by virtue of clinical autonomy can also be translated into expenditure figures, so in effect clinicians make not just medical decisions but also financial ones. Hunter comments: 'Getting a grip on the freedom enjoyed by clinicians and holding them to account for the expenditure they incur is seen as the last unmanaged frontier of the NHS' (Hunter 1994: 6). Significantly, Hunter adds that attempts to manage doctors' activities may not be successful unless time and effort are devoted to 'developing a managerial consciousness' among doctors, and unless there is 'an understanding of the doctor's world and culture' (ibid.: 12).

Essential elements of 'the doctor's world and culture' can be gleaned from the previous chapter in terms of the ideas, influences and conditions that gave rise to modern medicine. As Chapter 2 makes clear, a significant part of the medical model is the technological imperative, the ability and the requirement to intervene to produce a positive change in the body. The development of modern medicine is also crucially linked to ideas that emerged during **the Enlightenment** and this commitment to the principle of improving human welfare, combined with the Hippocratic oath, means that a doctor's first commitment has always been to the patient, or so it is argued. It is hardly surprising, then, that attempts to influence the behaviour of clinicians have been resisted. An analysis of the response of doctors to the introduction of the NHS in 1948 is evidence of this resistance. Doctors were willing to become employees of the NHS and wanted to retain their right to carry out work in the **private sector**. To this day general practitioners remain independent contractors who do work on behalf of the NHS but do not formally work *for* the NHS. Some attempts are being made to introduce salaried general practitioners – partly to ensure the availability of services in particularly deprived areas, but also to gain some influence over the activities of doctors.

It is important to note that restrictions on the activities of doctors have largely been intended to get to grips with the cost implications of their decision making, rather than to place restrictions on their professional autonomy. However, two regulatory bodies have been established in the UK in recent years – the National Institute for Clinical Excellence (NICE) in England and Wales, and NHS Quality Improvement Scotland (NHS QIS) – both of which rule on which drugs should be prescribed by the NHS. The roles of these organisations are principally to end what has been described as 'postcode prescribing', where local health boards (health authorities in England and Wales) make independent decisions about whether or not a specific drug can be prescribed within their area. NICE, for example, recommended the prescribing of Arecipt, a drug for the treatment of Alzheimer's disease. The decision was made on the basis of clinical effectiveness rather than purely on cost-effectiveness. The prescribing practices, however, of health authorities and health boards vary to such a degree that some patients will not have access to Arecipt.

The *clinical method*, the process that takes us from diagnosis to prognosis and treatment, remains very much intact. This should neither surprise nor, for the most part, alarm us, for the vast majority of clinical judgements are reasonable and bring about positive changes in the patient. However, some decisions can lead to negative effects on the patient, some are based on assumptions rather than on medical 'fact', while others are made without clear evidence to support them.

Medical harm: iatrogenesis

The first basis on which we can question the power of clinical freedom is in terms of its iatrogenic effects. The concept of **iatrogenesis**, associated with Illich, means 'doctor-caused illness', that is to say, harm would not have been caused *without* the medical intervention. Illich argues that the 'damage done by medicine to the health of the individuals and populations is very significant' (Illich 1993). This is referred to as 'clinical' iatrogenesis and Illich cites drug therapies, doctors or hospitals as the cause of harm. A second aspect is 'cultural' iatrogenesis, which denotes a dependence on medicine to cure and to care for. Illich argues that cultural iatrogenesis means that people no longer take responsibility for their own health problems and the diagnosis of their symptoms. Illich asserts that 'medical practice sponsors sickness … reinforcing a morbid society that encourages people to become consumers of curative, preventative, industrial and environmental medicine' (1993: 158). The result of this dependency is a situation of 'medical nemesis',

The **clinical method** refers to the process that begins with diagnosis and leads to a prognosis and subsequent treatment.

Iatrogenesis literally means harm caused by doctors. In its most literal sense it refers to the harmful consequences of medical intervention. Illich also uses the concept to draw our attention to our cultural dependence on medicine and medical practitioners, such that we do not seek alternative explanations or alternative remedics for ill health.

where the harm caused by medicine is difficult to eliminate except by recourse to further medical intervention, which in itself results in further harm. Illich paints a picture of an inevitable decline into an increasingly unhealthy world, where the provision of health care ultimately has a negative effect on our well-being.

Question

Think of your own examples of instances where medical intervention has had negative effects. What examples can you think of?

A balanced account of the harm resulting from health care would also, clearly, have to take into account positive developments in medicine. Hardley (1998) characterised the 1950s and 1960s as a period of great optimism about the potential of medicine to cure and care for people, and evidences this with reference to mass vaccination programmes that eradicated diseases such as polio and smallpox. At one end of the spectrum medicine can save and prolong life through radical interventions such as organ transplants, while at the more mundane end of the spectrum the symptoms of minor ailments such as headaches and menstrual pain can be eliminated by readily available pain relief. It is hardly surprising, therefore, that lay people may have a sense of dependency on medicine. Compared to people's experiences of health in the past, our own ill health may well seem trivial. Giddens comments that a glance at those experiences 'provides graphic evidence of the level to which illness and the prospect of an early death haunted the lives of individuals in the eighteenth century. Infectious diseases were rampant and the ordinary person suffered from a range of chronic complaints which many of us in modern social conditions would find intolerable' (Giddens 1997: 47–8).

In the eighteenth century in particular, deadly fevers – contemporaries called them 'spotted', 'miliary', 'hectic', 'malignant', etc. – struck down hundreds of thousands, young and old alike, while the so called 'new' diseases gained ground – some crippling such as rickets; some fatal, such as tuberculosis. Today's minor nuisance, like flu, was yesterday's killer. 'The Hooping Cough is yet with us', wrote George Crabbe in 1829, 'and many children die of it'. And all this against a backdrop of endemic maladies, such as malaria and infantile diarrhoea, and a Pandora's box of other infections (dysentery, scarlatina, measles, etc.) that commonly proved fatal, above all to infants, to say nothing of the 101 other pains, eruptions, swellings, ulcers, scrofula and wasting conditions, not least the agonizing stone and the proverbial gout, which threatened livings and livelihoods, and all too often life itself. (From L. Porter and L. Porter, 'Sickness and health in premodern England', repr. in Giddens 1997: 55)

The above discussion illustrates one strand of thinking which is critical of clinical autonomy on the basis of the harm resulting from medical intervention. The second level on which one can question the dominance of clinical autonomy is that clinical decisions are sometimes made on the basis of assumptions and beliefs rather than on scientific, objective grounds.

Fact or fiction? The making of medical decisions

Links

Chapter 2 provides a detailed account of the 'scientific' basis of the practice of medicine.

The previous chapter highlighted the extent to which the medical model is based on a commitment to scientific methods and empirical evidence, both of which suggest a high degree of objectivity. Critics of the medical model, however, have suggested that medicine is also the product of its social and cultural environments and, as such, is bound to reflect values dominant in **society**. Historically, the treatment of female patients provides a useful illustration of the extent to which medical categories reflect broader social and cultural values. Medicine does more than simply describe sets of symptoms; it may also create certain types of behaviour by applying a label to describe and categorise. According to Lupton (1996: 57) medicine can be seen as a 'moral exercise ... used to define normality, punish deviance and maintain social order'. A historical example of such a 'moral exercise' is **hysteria**.

James (1994) provides a detailed account of hysteria, its symptoms and remedies, from Greek theories of the womb's tendency to move around the body, to eighteenth-century theories of hysteria as a demonstration of the greater delicacy of women, particularly celibate women. Such ideas clearly resonated with ideas dominant at the time about women's essential differences from men. According to Turner (1994), descriptions of hysteria were linked to ideas about the subordination of women in so far as women were seen as 'naturally' frail and emotional. It had frequently been noted that the women who were most likely to experience hysteria (James 1994: 80) were unmarried and, therefore, seen as either sexually inactive or as sexually active but in an inappropriate manner. Neither celibacy nor unlicensed sexual activity was seen as conducive to physical or good mental health. The remedy for hysterical behaviour was, therefore, marriage and reproduction. It is important to remember that the eighteenth and nineteenth centuries are

Hysteria is the name of a 'disease' once associated with the movement of the womb around the body but later described as a disease of the nervous system. The symptoms of hysteria were described as weeping, fainting and a general malaise (James 1994).

associated with the beginnings of the modern women's movement, with its demand, for example, for equal access to education. Coincidentally, hysteria just happened to be diagnosed among women whose sexuality was not expressed 'normally', according to the prevailing values of the time, through marriage and child-bearing, and among women who attempted to pursue their education and careers. Turner writes that it was 'the absence of normal sexual activity designed to bring about reproduction which was associated in medical **discourse** with the prominence of hysteria' (Turner 1994: 84). The diagnosis of hysteria was linked not just with maintaining women's health but also with maintaining a specific pattern of gendered social relationships.

This chapter has established the ways in which medical power and knowledge can be used in positive and negative ways. The concept of clinical autonomy suggests that 'doctor knows best'. The preceding discussion has sought to highlight the specific nature of this professional dominance with examples such as the NHS reforms of the late 1980s and early 1990s when government attempted to rein in the power of the clinician. Two further examples, the concept of iatrogenesis and hysteria, were discussed to illustrate that clinical autonomy can be used to further ends other than to enhance the well-being of the patient. However, it might be argued that these are rather extreme examples, and that for the most part medicine does enhance health and well-being. Underpinning this line of argument is a strong belief that medicine is essentially a benign practice and that its ultimate function is to care for rather than to control. The following discussion challenges this idea by examining further the degree to which medicine is a disciplinary practice as much as a caring one.

3.2 Public health: the morality of everyday life

Links

The moralistic element of medicine was introduced in Chapter 2.

The previous discussion of **the medical model of health** draws our attention to the ways in which that model embraces issues relating to lifestyles and choice. 'Public health' refers to those areas of health and disease shared by the population in general and which are seen to be amenable to preventative intervention. Strategies to tackle public health cover more than simply medical techniques and have included measures to address housing problems, for example, and to ensure the supply of clean water and adequate sanitation. Contemporary definitions of public health have tended to take as their object the environment, including social, psychological and physical elements (Peterson 1997: 192–3).

There are four significant points that arise from these public health initiatives. First, the at-risk category embraces most people. Health and the practice of medicine, therefore, no longer embrace only those who are diseased but now encompass even those who are well. Second, public health appears to be concerned with the regulation and control of individual bodies. Lupton (1995: 30) argues that controlling and preventing the spread of disease has largely involved confining bodies and controlling their movements. Third, over and above the control and regulation of individuals is the regulation of the social body. Many of the facts and figures presented throughout this book are themselves a product of the public health movement and, in particular, of attempts to 'map' the spread of disease and its distribution within the population. Epidemiology involves the recording of information, 'constant record-taking, measuring and reporting back to a system of government agencies' (Lupton 1995: 31). Increasingly our risk of disease becomes understood in terms of statistical probability calculated for us by experts. Finally, what emerges from an analysis of public health initiatives is a sense of what is pathological (diseased) and what is normal health and behaviour. The latter is often understood as what is statistically average. Seale points to this tendency and highlights its implications in terms of the association of normality with what *ought* to be the case (Seale 1998: 105).

Surveillance refers to a form of scrutiny and observation but one that does not necessarily depend directly on the physical proximity of the watcher and the watched. Instead, subtle forms of surveillance are said to characterise modern society, typified by the tendency of individuals to act in ways that they think they 'ought' to.

Links

Chapter 7, sections 7.1 and 7.2, provides a discussion of the body as a site of control and regulation, not only for health professionals but for individuals as well.

The control and regulation of disease

The act of collecting information, analysing that information and calculating 'risk' suggests that knowledge is being used as a form of power and influence. At one end of the spectrum, this form of power could be described as 'disciplinary' (for example, confining infected bodies to their homes), or at the very least as 'directional' (for example, directing us towards healthy eating practices). The work of Foucault leads us to the conclusion that the modern period is associated with subtle forms of power, control and regulation. The best illustration of this form of power is the panopticon – a construction containing a central observation tower around which other buildings are placed and into which the occupant of the central tower can see. The occupants of the outlying buildings are not afforded the same opportunity and do not know when or if they are being watched. The aim of this system of **surveillance** is to ensure that this state of uncertainty is transformed into self-surveillance. Such a system is in stark contrast to sovereign forms of power, exemplified by sixteenth- and seventeenth-century monarchs. Under their regimes, Seale argues, power was manifest in rather more obvious and brutal forms, principally through 'physical coercion and public punishment for wrongdoing' (Seale 1998: 105). Public acts of punishment were a reminder of the power of the monarch and it was the act of punishment that marked an individual as an 'out law'. In contrast, disciplinary power 'operated by constructing and promoting, with the aid of statistical information, particular definitions of normality. From being coerced to follow the will of the king, citizens learned to survey themselves as bearers of normality' (ibid.: 105).

Question

Can you identify any incidents in your own life where you have been assessed for 'normal functioning'?

A specific example of surveillance and self-surveillance can be found in the case of screening for cervical cancer. Research carried out by McKie suggests that in this instance 'screening is both creating and reinforcing a surveillance of women's sexual lives and health' (McKie 1995: 441). As the above discussion describes, screening involves not only uncovering infection but also identifying groups at risk. In the case of cervical cancer, treatment is not confined to women with cervical cancer but includes those women identified as having pre-cancerous cells that might develop into cervical cancer at a later stage. An additional complication with this form of screening is that there are difficulties in establishing the causes of cervical cancer and thus there is a further difficulty in differentiating between those women who might consider themselves normal and those who might be most at risk. For this reason the at-risk category essentially embraces all women. Failure to recognise your own at-risk status is viewed in negative terms. 'Women are encouraged to attend on a regular basis and those who do not are often considered by health care workers to be irresponsible, feckless and non-compliers' (McKie 1995: 445).

McKie highlights the extent to which much of the surveillance carried out by the medical profession on behalf of the state is of behaviours that are believed to lead to the spread of the disease. Despite the causes of cervical cancer being unclear, many researchers maintain that the human papilloma virus HPV, which can be transmitted through sexual intercourse, is to be found in the majority of cancers. As McKie points out, this in itself raises the question of the causes of HPV and a number of factors are said to place women at greater risk. These include age, heterosexual intercourse, lower age at first intercourse and smoking status. It is, therefore, not just the cervix itself that is subject to surveillance but types of behaviour, many of which – such as sexual intercourse at an early age and sexual promiscuity – have negative connotations. To receive a positive result for a cervical cancer may stigmatise the woman as someone who 'sleeps around' (McKie 1995: 449). In this instance it is possible to argue that screening does not simply describe what is the case (the number of women with cervical cancer) but has implications for what ought to be by suggesting a link between stigmatised behaviours and the causes of the disease. Screening for cervical cancer, therefore, carries with it certain normative assumptions about how women ought to behave, and this extends to the assumption that all women are heterosexual. This assumption is especially significant since many practitioners use the 'smear' as an opportunity to talk to women about other health issues, principally contraception and sexual health, again based on the same assumption of exclusively heterosexual experiences.

The preceding discussion raises the issue of medicine as a moral discourse regulating various aspects of our lives. An important aspect of this regulation is surveillance of our own behaviour, convinced as we are of the morality of what we are required to do when, for example, submitting ourselves to screening for diseases. Surveillance is a form of power that does not physically constrain or persecute people but apparently gives people the freedom of taking responsibility for their own health and well-being. As Seale comments, concepts of normality become internalised 'so that under disciplinary power, people constantly monitor themselves for signs of pathology. Thus people draw upon a widespread knowledge of what it is to be sane, healthy and good, and of their opposites, madness, disease and criminality' (Seale 1998: 106).

One conclusion that can be drawn is that the power of clinicians does not so much reside in the person as in the profession. Such conclusions are well recorded within the sociology of health. Parsons' concept of **the sick role** is a clear example of a model that not only accepts that there is inequality in the clinician/patient relationship, but that this actually benefits both parties. The following discussion examines the continuing power of the medical profession.

1. Legitimises withdrawal from a range of 'normal' obligations, such as paid work.
2. A person cannot get well without the intervention of a medical professional.
3. People have a social obligation to get well as soon as possible. This is the only basis upon which legitimate access to the 'sick role' is granted.
4. Care has to be provided by a competent medical practitioner.
5. The doctor/patient relationship is characterised by neutrality.
6. In return for compliance with the 'sick role' the patient is provided with medical care.
7. Doctors have the right to diagnose, examine and treat patients.

FIGURE 3.2   *Parsons' concept of the sick role*
Source: adapted from Turner (1994: 46)

3.3 'The latter-day 'resurrectionists': the continuing power of the medical profession

Links

A description of the functionalist approach is available in Chapter 1.

Parsons' functionalist account of the sick role lays out the roles, responsibilities and rights of patients and practitioners based on an assumption of a consensus between the two parties, ultimately beneficial to both (see Figure 3.2).

A number of criticisms of the concept of the sick role are particularly relevant to this discussion about the power of the medical profession. According to Turner, one major area of criticism has been Parsons' assumption that the doctor/patient relationship is 'complementary and functional' (Turner 1994: 46). Not only does sociological research suggest that patients may be well informed and, therefore, questioning of the treatment provided, but it suggests that the power of the practitioner is not always used for the benefit of the patient. Certainly, arguments such as these have been used to justify the practice of clinical autonomy. The NHS reforms of the 1980s and 1990s challenged the undisputed power of clinicians with the introduction of the principle of general management. It was not difficult for critics of the reforms to argue that it could only be practitioners who had the best interests of the patients at heart since it was practitioners, not managers, who had direct contact with them. Counter-arguments centred on questioning whether practitioners could also use clinical autonomy to safeguard their own professional interests. Resources might be used to research a particular disease, for example, with ultimate benefit to the patient. However, resources for research might also further an individual clinician's career in so far as it enabled someone to pursue a particular interest and add to their reputation and knowledge.

Example

A contemporary example of the tendency of the population to contest the power of the medical profession is the current resistance to the MMR triple vaccine. Despite reassurances by the medical profession that the triple vaccine is safe, large sections of the general public remain sceptical.

Links

The concept of the sociological imagination is detailed in Chapter 1. Chapter 2, section 2.4, provides a detailed discussion of the clinical gaze.

To fully understand the nature of the relationship between the practitioner and the patient it is necessary to employ the **sociological imagination** to uncover what lies behind the obvious. Within **sociology**, there is a long tradition of acknowledging that the possession of knowledge is a form of power. Such an approach is evident in the work of Foucault and the concept of the **clinical gaze**. The 'gaze' not only reveals a specific way of 'seeing' the body (or the insides of the body); with it comes a whole vocabulary by which to know and interpret the body. This specialist knowledge has the effect of excluding other, alternative explanations of the body and disease. The work of Becker (1974) and the labelling tradition also allows us to explore how knowledge is used as a form of social control. A central tenet of labelling **theory** is the acceptance of the social construction of knowledge. In other words, meanings are not fixed but are the outcome of a process of definition, a process in which some groups and individuals have considerably more say than others. Within the labelling tradition, deviance has 'no consistent unitary content or essence' (Turner 1994: 73). It is possible to interpret medical knowledge as a form of labelling in so far as diagnostic categories are ways of describing and categorising behaviour. It is useful to reflect on an example of research used in the opening chapter. There we outlined Rosenhan's (1973) work, 'On being sane in insane places', which concluded that diagnostic categories were social constructs with which it was possible to both describe and create 'madness'.

The making of life-and-death decisions

The ability to diagnose, recommend and carry out treatment represents a distinctive form of power. Simple examples of this power are evident in relation to pregnancy and death. Pregnancy may be evident to the mother-to-be and those around here, but it awaits 'official' confirmation by the medical profession. Again, it may be clear to others that death has taken place but it is not for them to confirm that. Illich argues that the degree of control exercised by the medical professional is extensive: it 'starts with the monthly prenatal check-up when he decides if and how the foetus shall be born; it ends with his decision to abandon further resuscitation' (Illich, cited in Harvey 1997: 719).

Reproductive technology involves new techniques of surveillance and examination, such as ultrasound and foetal monitoring, that make the woman and the unborn child 'visible' in a way that turns them both into objects and subjects of medical, legal and state intervention. Doyal (1994) calls the foetus the 'newly discovered second patient' and describes situations where doctors seek court orders to protect the best interests of their 'new' patients.

The legal and medical professions, it is argued, are the 'managers' of death. Harvey asserts that the medical dominance of death is reflected in the mirroring of medical images of death in the popular consciousness. She argues that 'the "straight green line" on the oscilloscope has become a compelling late twentieth-century image of death, while the electronic alarm signal has replaced the (organic) death rattle in popular consciousness' (1997: 725). Harvey suggests that in situations where therapeutic intervention has reached its limits and there is no improvement in the patient's condition, clinicians may consider 'withdrawal of active support' (ibid.: 724). Such support is reduced on a gradual basis, Harvey's research suggests, in order to mimic a natural, gradual death. There are said to be specific benefits to this approach. In the first instance, it allows relatives of the patient to come to terms with the imminent death of a loved one. Second, death is less dramatic, less like pointing a gun at someone, as one of the interviewed consultants, suggested.

Question

Prior to the rise of the medical profession who would have been actively involved in the diagnosis of death?

The making of 'end-of-life decisions' is clearly fraught with medical, technological, legal and ethical considerations. With the power to save and prolong life comes the onerous power to end it. Wade, a consultant and professor in neurological disability, explores the specific example of patients in a permanent vegetative state (Wade 2001). Permanent vegetative state is characterised by Wade in the following manner (2001: 352):

1   The patient shows no behavioural evidence of awareness of self or environment.
2   There is brain damage, usually of known cause, consistent with the diagnosis.
3   There are no reversible causes present, and
4   At least six (usually 12) months have passed since the onset of PVS.

A number of ethical issues are raised not just by the decision to end a life but, Wade suggests, by the diagnosis itself. He suggests that the diagnosis is not certain and there is no standard test to assess levels of awareness. The actual decision to withdraw feeding is fraught with legal and ethical issues. For example, treating a patient who may be regarded as 'non-sentient' raises questions about how to maintain that person's dignity and privacy. Committing resources to the care of people in a permanent vegetative state raises issues about the rationing of scarce health resources: 'is it equitable to allocate substantial scarce resources to someone who is unaware of their situation and will not recover awareness?' (Wade 2001: 352). Wade recognises that the issue raises questions outside the remit of individual clinicians, and argues that one solution might be to take into consideration the interests of other parties, 'and to use a full ethical accounting procedure' (ibid.). The suggestions are interesting, if only because they seek to share out the responsibility for decision making in relation to the ending of life.

Decision making relating to the ending of life is complex and demonstrates both the actual and the potential power that clinicians have to make decisions. In the light of technological advancement they are increasingly being faced with decisions that might appear to be purely clinical but are also ethical and legal. While the death of a patient might be seen as a failure in terms of the medical profession's ability to maintain life, death itself provides important information and 'resources' that can save other lives and advance medical knowledge. One of the key factors that allowed the development of clinical medicine was the ability to examine the corpse and to learn from this. Thus pathology plays an important part in developing medical knowledge. Clinicians no longer have to rely upon 'resurrectionists' to supply them with bodies, since social and cultural taboos about the use of dead bodies have largely been eroded. It is a legal requirement in the case of sudden or violent death for a post-mortem to take place and for tissue to be retained as evidence. Many thousands of people carry organ donor cards and the medical profession talks openly about the 'harvesting' of organs for the purpose of transplants.

Despite a general acceptance of the use of dead bodies for teaching and research purposes and the desirability of 'harvesting' organs in order to prolong the life of others, revelations about the extent and nature of the retention of such material has caused national outrage. When it emerged in 1999 that various organs from children treated at the Alder Hey Hospital in Liverpool had been removed and retained without the knowledge or consent of parents, there were calls to government to ensure that this would not happen again. While there was widespread condemnation of these practices by other clinicians, the case, nevertheless, represented a dilemma for the medical profession. It was important to be seen to act ethically and with the consent of relatives, but at the same time there was a necessity to secure an adequate supply of human tissue to continue research.

> Professor Gordon McVie, director general of the Cancer Research Campaign, told the *BMJ [British Medical Journal]* that, although researchers remained 'extremely sensitive to the issue of patient consent', it was unreasonable to expect scientists to list every use a tissue sample might be put to.
>
> 'It's impossible to predict everything you are going to do. There are 3,000 genes linked to breast cancer. Are you going to list them all on a consent form?'
>
> Professor McVie expressed concern that plans to create banks of excised tumour tissue to aid cancer research could be put at risk if all collection of tissue was restricted. (Hunter 2001: 322)

Liam Donaldson, Chief Medical Officer in England and Wales, advised that informed consent should be sought rather than simple 'lack of objection' and that consent forms should contain 'details of the tissue and organs to be retained, the uses to which they might be put, and the agreed length of time for retention' (Hunter 2001: 322). Confusion had arisen in particular about the ambiguous use of the word 'tissue', which to lay people suggested small, insignificant parts of organs or blood vessels. In contrast, clinicians used the term as a catch-all category to include substantial body parts such as the heart. The characteristics of the medical model outlined in the first chapter are a reminder of the 'mechanical' metaphor for the workings and parts which make up the human body. It is possible to argue on the basis of the Alder Hey scandal that the medical model, the clinical gaze, has the effect of dehumanising the body and obscuring the ability of those involved to appreciate the significance of the 'whole' body for family and friends.

Links

Chapter 2 provides an overview of the significance of the postmortem for the development of medical knowledge.

Patient
May have pre-existing statement of wishes.
May have wished to donate organs.
May have had strong beliefs (religious or otherwise)
May or may not be experiencing emotions
May have strong beliefs.

Ward staff
May have emotional interests in patient or family
May have strong beliefs.

Organisation funding care
May wish to allocate resources differently

Relatives (and friends)
May have a financial interest (will or settlement)
May have other legal interests.
May have emotional or other stressful experiences
May be ignoring children or others.

Organisation giving care
May have financial interests (positive or negative)
May have political or public relationship interests

Society
May wish to preserve sanctity of life.
May wish to avoid 'slippery slope'.
May support different allocation of resources.

FIGURE 3.3   *Permament vegetative state: interested parties and their interests (Wade 2001)*

Conclusion

This chapter has examined the extent and nature of the power of the medical profession in relation to clinical autonomy, public health and contemporary examples of decisions made about ending life and retaining human organs for research. Much of the apparent power of clinicians rests on the possession of a specialist body of knowledge that provides a justification for the exclusion of others from the process of decision making. This conclusion does not deny the obvious benefits of medical intervention but seeks to draw attention to the implications of the use of power.

Public health programmes such as mass screening have played a central role in the elimination of diseases such as polio, but it is also clear from the examples discussed above that such programmes are underpinned by a strong sense of what people 'ought' to do.

It is possible, therefore, to conclude that public health is at least directional, if not a form of disciplinary power. Contemporary examples of the practice of medicine, such as the Alder Hey scandal, underline the fact that medicine is open to criticism.

SUMMARY POINTS

- Medicine's power is based on a specialist knowledge base and clinical autonomy.
- Medical decisions are not always based on evidence.
- Critics, such as Illich, point to how medicine can cause harm.
- Public health programmes can also act as a form of social control.

The following chapter considers the basis upon which such criticisms have been made and looks at possible alternatives to current orthodox medical knowledge and practice.

Case study

Callum has been in a permanent vegative state for three months, following a car crash. There are no signs to indicate that he will ever gain consciousness again, leaving his parents in a state of confusion and misery. His body appears unmarked, undamaged but with no hope of recovery. At the age of 18 he was a fit and healthy young man, but now it appears that his life is over. His parents are reluctant to do anything that will end his life. As long as he stays this way he is at least not lost to them, and yet there can be no more engagement with him.

Using the series of questions set by Wade in his 'Interested Parties' concept (pp. 47–9 above), analyse this situation and reflect upon how ending this life would impact on all the people involved, both family and care providers.

Taking your studies further

This chapter will have helped you understand many of the key terms, concepts, theories and debates relating to medical power and knowledge. Listed below are journal articles and books that will provide deeper and more detailed discussions of the points raised in this chapter. You will also find what is available on the companion website. This offers downloads of relevant material, plus links to useful websites in addition to podcasts and other features.

Recommended reading

Petersen, A.R. and Lupton, D. (2000) *The New Public Health: Discourses, Knowledges, Strategies.* London: Sage.

Journal articles

Harvey, J. (1997) 'The technological regulation of death: with reference to the technological regulation of birth', *Sociology*, 31 (4): 719–35.

Seymour, J.E. (2000) 'Negotiating natural death in intensive care', *Social Science and Medicine*, 51 (8): 1241–52.

Seymour, J.E. (1999) 'Revisiting medicalisation and "natural" death', *Social Science and Medicine*, 49 (5): 691–704.

On the companion website

Lee-Treweek, G. (2001) 'I'm not ill, it's just this back: osteopathic treatment, responsibility and back problems', *Health*, 5 (1): 31–49.

4

Challenging medical dominance

MAIN POINTS

- Medicine has encroached upon many aspects of life that were once considered normal or 'natural'. This is termed 'medicalisation'.
- One example of medicalisation is pregnancy and childbirth. Doctors and medical technology can challenge women's control and experiences of fertility.
- Alternative, or complementary, medicine is becoming increasingly popular, due to an increased individualism, disengagement with community and dissatisfaction with mainstream medicine.

KEY CONCEPTS

Complementary medicine, alternative medicine, reproductive technology, medicalisation.

Introduction

The previous chapter gave specific examples of medical power by exploring the concept of **clinical autonomy**, the morality implicit in public health messages, and medicine's continuing access to and control over the body. This chapter seeks to analyse the basis upon which critics have challenged that dominance. There are two major themes to be explored here. The first is that of the medical control and regulation of women's lives in the context of reproduction and **reproductive technology**. Feminist critiques of medicine are concerned not only with the numerical dominance of men in the profession in general as well as in specific areas such as acute services, but with challenging the values, beliefs and ideology associated with the **theory** and practice of medicine. The second theme to be examined is that of alternative or complementary therapies. Like the feminist critique of medicine, alternative perspectives represent a radical challenge to the most basic concepts and practices of western biomedicine.

Reproductive technology embraces a range of medical interventions (pharmaceutical and invasive), the purpose of which is either to promote or to prevent pregnancy. The concept of **medicalisation** is used to describe a tendency to explain behaviour and experiences in medical terms.

Links

See Chapter 3, section 3.1 for a related discussion of the concept of clinical autonomy.

4.1 'The miracle of life': the medical colonisation of reproduction

Feminist critiques of medicine challenge the way in which women's lives, principally in relation to reproduction, have been subject to the control of the medical profession, with women themselves seen as passive objects. The phrase *reproductive technology* refers not only to pregnancy and birth but also to the use of contraception and to assisted conception in the form of IVF, for example. Oakley suggests that reproduction embraces both the 'promotion of pregnancy' and the 'preventing of pregnancy' (Oakley 1987: 40). This type of control and regulation is representative of the degree to which women's lives are subject to **medicalisation**. Previous chapters have already made reference to the manner in which medical knowledge can be used as a form of power, and the extent to which the practice of medicine can be based on moral judgements rather than on scientific evidence. In relation to this discussion of reproduction it is particularly helpful to think about medicalisation as the way in which specific 'behaviours or conditions are given medical meanings and thus medical practice becomes the appropriate vehicle for their elimination or control' (Levinson 1998: 75). In this way, the apparently 'natural' process of reproduction is defined as a medical condition requiring 'expert' knowledge, treatment and intervention.

A significant aspect of the concept of medicalisation is the extent to which natural experiences are transformed into medical ones. Oakley provides historical evidence of how the experiences of pregnancy and childbirth were significantly changed by medical intervention. Prior to the widespread dominance of biomedicine, Oakley argues, the main healers in society were lay women. 'Childbirth occurred at home. There was no systematic medical care during pregnancy. Institutions grouping pregnant and labouring women as "patients" along with the sick did not exist' (Oakley 1987: 37). It was not until the eighteenth century that childbirth became increasingly technical and appropriated by male medical practitioners. The opportunity to study pregnancy and childbirth was facilitated by the use of hospitals to care for women.

Links

The medicalisation of death is dealt with in Chapter 3, section 3.3.

Similar themes emerge from Reissman's account of the medicalisation of childbirth in mid-nineteenth-century America. Like Oakley, Reissman argues that childbirth increasingly came to be seen as a technical problem, thus requiring the expert intervention of the medical profession within a suitable physical location, namely the hospital rather than the home. She suggests that this process of medicalisation resulted in a fundamental change to the nature of childbirth: 'the meaning of childbirth for women was transformed from a human experience to a medical technical problem' (Reissman 1992: 127). The emerging profession of obstetrics reached a position of dominance for a variety of social and medical reasons. Obstetricians were male, mainly white and middle-class, enjoying social and **class** dominance over the female, lower-class, and mainly immigrant midwives. Of particular importance, argues Reissman, was the ability of the emerging profession to convince both colleagues and the public that pregnancy required medical and technical intervention in order to reach a successful conclusion. Most significantly of all, mothers were seen as passive objects, knowing less about their own pregnancy than the medical expert.

Oakley suggests that this shift towards the definition of women as 'mindless mothers' emerged at the same time as the technological dominance of pregnancy (1987: 39). The notion of women as 'walking wombs' is clearly illustrated by the following conversation recorded by Oakley (ibid.: 46):

Patient It's the tightening I worry about.
Doctor It's normal in pregnancy. Your womb is supposed to tighten.
Patient I didn't have it with the other three.
Doctor Every pregnancy is different. Let's see you in one week.
 [Reading notes] You do seem to have put on a bit of weight.
Patient What does that mean?
Doctor It doesn't necessarily mean anything but you must take things easy.
Patient That's what my husband says. It's easy for men to say that.
Doctor You shouldn't blame us.
Patient I'm not blaming you. It's not your fault.
Doctor It's your set-up at home. You should have organised things better.
Patient Well, I've got three kids to look after.
Doctor Yes.

Oakley's **analysis** of the conversation is intended to illustrate the power dynamics implicit in the doctor–patient relationship. She argues that first the doctor dismisses the patient's understanding of her condition and the authority of his own knowledge is reaffirmed. Second, the conversation reveals the power the doctor possesses in terms of withholding information. The patient's weight is commented upon but the doctor does not reveal the significance of this fact. The conversation also reveals a general acceptance on the part of both the patient and the doctor of women's responsibility for childcare and housework. The patient herself is seen as being responsible for not taking things easy. Oakley concludes that the doctor is concerned primarily with the technical management of the pregnancy rather than with the real person coping with both her pregnancy and domestic responsibilities. 'The problem of pregnancy management as he has defined it discounts the importance of the whole person' (Oakley 1987: 47).

Feminist critics have questioned the reasoning behind the accepted ways of treating pregnancy and delivering babies. Doyal (1994) talks about potentially demeaning practices such as the shaving of pubic hair and the giving of enemas. Other commentators have questioned the need for the majority of births to take place in hospitals, suggesting that most labours are 'uneventful' and as such could take place in the woman's own home (Lupton 1995: 148). Removing pregnant women to the hospital environment suggests that pregnancy is an illness, and has the added disadvantage of placing women in an environment unknown to them at a time when they are particularly vulnerable (ibid.). Responses to such criticisms have come in two main forms: the development of a natural childbirth movement, and a change in the attitudes and practices of the medical profession itself. Natural childbirth is defined as childbirth with 'as little drug intervention as possible' (ibid.). The degree to which the medical profession has embraced a more 'natural' model of childbirth is subject to debate, but there is a growing recognition of the need to allow women to make informed choices about how and where they deliver.

Feminist critique can suggest that medicine and medical practitioners see women as objects and mindless mothers who play no part in deciding what kind of medical care they receive. What is perhaps lacking from this analysis is an appreciation that women have at times welcomed technological interventions and even benefited from them. Reissman argues that women 'participated in the medicalisation of childbirth for a complex set of reasons' (1992: 128). The principal reason was a desire to find relief from the pain and frequency of childbirth. The desire for pain relief was, Reissman comments, part of a change in social attitudes towards pregnancy, with childbirth no longer seen as 'a condition to be endured with fatalism and passivity' (ibid.: 129). An overall reduction in fertility rates, especially marked among the middle and upper classes, meant that the experience of birth was changing. The fact that women had fewer children resulted in increased anxiety about childbirth and a greater desire for the delivery to take place safely. In the broader context of medicalisation generally, Lupton reminds us that patients and doctors might well collude, effectively enhancing the medical dominance of the latter (Lupton 1995: 98). While medical power can be seen as 'disciplining' and controlling people's lives, it may well be true that people give themselves over to medical power voluntarily because of the apparent benefits that accrue.

Question

In terms of pregnancy and childbirth, what are the benefits of medical intervention?

Part of Oakley's critique of the medicalisation of pregnancy and childbirth is the failure of the medical profession to take into consideration the whole person. Instead, she argues, women are seen as 'mindless mothers' whose own experiences and knowledge of pregnancy are often ignored. An essential element of the concept of medicalisation can thus be understood as the transformation of human experiences into medical and technical ones. According to Oakley, the personal and social implications of medical treatment are rarely considered:

> It took some twenty years for the practitioners of obstetric ultrasound to wake up to the fact that seeing her foetus on the screen might change the way a woman felt about it. This elementary piece of wisdom has translated into technical paediatric language and the notion of prenatal mother–child bonding was born. (Oakley 1987: 52)

Links

Chapter 3 examines the ability of the medical profession to place the body, even in its inner workings, under surveillance.

In a similar vein, Lupton has considered how the procedure of genetic testing involves a new **discourse** of the body. It is impossible, Lupton suggests, to separate the technical aspects of genetic screening from its social and emotional implications. Part of the basis upon which people are persuaded of the necessity of undergoing such tests is an appeal to their emotions and anxieties about being a 'good' and responsible parent. Genetic screening provides a very different way of understanding the body; it becomes a collection of codes, like a machine-based system, that can only be interpreted by 'experts' (Lupton 1995). Lupton suggests that this particular discourse on the body has little meaning to lay people. Being told of your risk of passing on a genetically inherited disease in purely statistical terms can appear overly abstract and difficult to translate into the decision to carry on with or terminate the pregnancy. Lupton contrasts the 'abstract language of biomedicine' with the 'individualised narratives' provided by the parents themselves (ibid.: 152).

Assisted conception

The medicalisation of pregnancy and childbirth has a relatively long history but medical dominance is increasingly interpreted in terms of the ability to create life in the various forms of assisted conception. The following discussion has two main strands: first, an examination of the social, ethical and cultural implications of assisted conception and, second, a consideration of the implications of the medical dominance of women's lives. The preceding chapter outlined the scope and power of medicine in relation to its ability to prolong and enhance life. It was noted that while science provides the means to transform our lives, it does not answer the question of whether or not such interventions should take place. Ethical debates about the use of biomedicine are nowhere more acute than around the use and potential of assisted conception. Debates about assisted conception necessarily go beyond helping those people who are unable to conceive naturally, and embrace complex arguments about its use (and potential misuse), such as the storing of human embryos.

The use of assisted conception brings into sharp relief the question of who is the parent of the child, and under what circumstances. In normal circumstances, the parentage of a child seems a simple matter. This is true in the case of the mother (there can be little dispute about who has given birth) but slightly more problematic in the case of the father who, it can be argued, does not know beyond doubt that he is the father of the child, without the aid of blood tests. Parentage, however, is more than simply providing the genetic material to produce a child: it also involves the social roles and responsibilities associated with raising that child. As Smart (1996) has commented, 'motherhood' is more than a biological relationship; simply giving birth does not result in 'motherhood' or 'mothering'. However, with assisted conception it is possible to extend the notion of 'mother'. Lupton comments that we can refer to someone as an 'egg mother', 'birth mother', 'surrogate mother', 'legal mother' or 'adoptive mother'. Similarly, sperm donation raises the question of whether the donor could enjoy the status of 'father' (Lupton 1995: 156). The Human Fertilisation and Embryology Act of 1990 attempts to circumvent this complex debate by providing what Franklin describes as a technical definition of 'mother'. The Act describes a mother as 'the woman who is carrying or has carried a child as a result of the placing in her of an embryo or of sperm and eggs' (Franklin 1997: 226).

Links

For a related discussion on the ability of the medical profession to make life-or-death decisions, see Chapter 3, section 3.3.

The use of assisted conception raises a further complex question about who should have access to those techniques and enjoy the experience and status of a parent. Debates about access are only partly about the resources to fund such techniques; perhaps more importantly these debates also centre upon a person's (usually a couple's) desire and suitability to parent. According to Franklin (1997), the desire to parent is seen as a 'natural' impulse. The Warnock Report (1985), set up to debate ethical issues arising from techniques of assisted conception, argued that for many childless couples the social pressures to parent were very significant. Being childless is often seen as a 'failure' to fulfil convention (Franklin 1997: 91). Franklin cites the authors of *The Infertility Handbook* who argue that there is a biological impulse to reproduce: 'Call it a cosmic spark or spiritual fulfilment, biological need or human destiny – the desire for a family rises unbidden from our genetic souls' (Bellina and Wilson 1986: xv; cited in Franklin 1997: 91). It is equally clear, however, that this desire to have a child has to be understood within a social and cultural context and in the case of many western countries this is within the framework of the family, most commonly understood as a heterosexual (married) couple. Such a definition excludes both single women and lesbians who, presumably, are not thought to possess the same biological desire to reproduce. Patrick Steptoe, one of the pioneers of assisted conception techniques, argued that such women should be excluded on the basis that for them to have children would be unnatural and morally wrong (Franklin 1997: 92).

Question

There are many restrictions placed on who may parent via assisted conception. What would your reaction be if similar restrictions were placed on parents who can conceive without medical intervention?

Access to techniques of assisted conception is, therefore, restricted on social and moral grounds. Doyal argues that access to reproductive technology is thus only possible with what she refers to as the tacit or explicit agreement of the medical profession.

For Castells, as for many commentators, the advent of reproductive technologies such as assisted conception represents women's 'growing control over the timing and frequency of child bearing' (Castells 1997: 135). For others, such as Porter (1990), this optimism is misguided, as access to such techniques, she argues, is only achieved via the gatekeepers of services, namely the medical profession. Porter highlights the extent to which developments in assisted conception have meant the medicalisation of conception as well as of contraception and childbirth. The end result is the exercise of control over 'means of reproduction – access to procedures, technology, information and so on – and thereby controls over women's bodies and ultimately their lives' (Porter 1990: 185).

Porter's research indicated that medical professionals worked with 'ideal types' in relation to the provision of specific methods of contraception. The ideal patient for sterilisation was 'a woman in her early thirties, happily married with two or three children. The ideal type depo provera patient was a woman in her early thirties with a large number of unwanted pregnancies, not in a stable relationship and living in local authority housing in a poor part of the city' (Porter 1990: 195). The significance of these ideal types lies in the way in which doctors were reluctant to offer alternative forms of contraception to women who did not fit their ideal type.

Oakley (1987) has noted that in relation to pregnancy and childbirth women largely appear as passive objects and recipients of care. A similar tendency to describe women in passive terms – here as recipients of embryos – is noticeable in relation to assisted conception. Lupton highlights a contrast: 'male scientists and doctors are commonly portrayed as active, expert and rational, the "producers" and "fathers" of "test-tube babies", while women are represented as desperate for children, passive, reacting emotionally to their chance to experience the joys of desired motherhood' (Lupton 1995: 157). According to Franklin, descriptions of IVF treatment tend to underplay the role of would-be parents, in particular that of the mother, and to emphasise the creative power of medical technology (Franklin 1997: 103). An unquestioning commitment on the part of the hopeful parents to the technological processes involved is ensured by seeking to portray the medical profession as simply lending a helping hand in an otherwise completely 'natural' process (ibid.). Franklin describes initial accounts of IVF as oversimplified – omitting, for example, to provide an accurate representation of the failure rate. The only agency referred to is that of the 'invisible hand of technology' which facilitates conception (ibid.: 104). Medicine itself has brought forth the 'miracle of life'.

The preceding discussion has sought to illustrate both the dominance of the medical profession and the challenges made to this position by feminist critics. In the following discussion, a further dimension of the challenge to biomedicine is introduced in the form of alternative therapies.

4.2 Challenging the dominance of the biomedical model: alternative therapies

Alternative, or complementary, therapies embrace many philosophies and methods but collectively represent a challenge to the concepts of health and disease articulated in the medical model. This part of the discussion begins by defining what is meant by 'alternative' practices and provides specific examples.

In their broadest sense, the terms **alternative medicine** and *complementary medicine* can be used to describe any practices that fall outside the boundaries of conventional medicine. West (1993) acknowledges that it is problematic to try and define such a diverse body of practices but offers the possibility of categorising different types. The main categories are identified as physical, psychological and paranormal. She suggests a further distinction between practices that demand a high level of training and those she describes as virtually 'do-it-yourself'. For others the principal distinction between 'alternative' and biomedicine is the former's 'holistic' emphasis. Saks suggests that in 'orthodox' medicine, the overwhelming emphasis is on the physical, with the mind and the spirit 'still typically regarded as relatively peripheral to health care' (Saks 1998: 198). In contrast and despite their apparent diversity, most alternative therapies deal 'with the unity of the mind, body and spirit' (ibid.). The following are examples of two alternative approaches to understanding health and illness.

Two examples of alternative practices

Homoeopathy is an effective and scientific system of healing which assists the natural tendency of the body to heal itself. It assumes that all symp toms of ill health are expressions of disharmony within the whole person and that it is the patient who needs treatment not the disease. *Source*: www.apothecary.co.uk

Acupuncture is medical treatment that can relieve symptoms of some physical and psychological conditions and may encourage the patient's body to heal and repair itself, if it is able to do so. Acupuncture stimulates the nerves in skin and muscle, and can produce a variety of effects. We know that it increases the body's release of natural painkillers – endorphin and serotonin – in the pain pathways of both the spinal cord and the brain. This modifies the way pain signals are received.

But acupuncture does much more than reduce pain, and has a beneficial effect on health. Patients often notice an improved sense of well-being after treatment. Modern research shows that acupuncture can affect most of the body's systems – the nervous system, muscle tone, hormone outputs, circulation, antibody production and allergic responses, as well as the respiratory, digestive, urinary and reproductive systems.
Source: www.medical-acupuncture.co.uk

Alternative medicine embraces any medical practice that falls outside the boundaries of conventional medicine. Some commentators use the term 'complementary medicine' to imply that non-conventional medicine can be used in conjunction with western biomedicine rather than as a radical alternative.

The professional marginalisation of alternative medicine

An important element of alternative medicine's status as 'other' and different from orthodox medicine rests on the different conceptualisations of the relationship between the mind, body and spirit. A second and equally important element of the status of alternative practices is their institutional and professional marginalisation in relation to orthodox medicine. Chapter 3 examined the extent of the professional dominance of biomedicine, a dominance powerfully signalled by the illegality of other occupational groups carrying out tasks for which medical practitioners alone are state registered. Surgical procedures, for example, are the exclusive province of doctors. Other professionals, such as nurses, may observe and assist but not carry out the procedure itself. Saks (1994) argues that this professional dominance was enhanced by the establishment of the NHS in 1948 because the only form of health care accessible, 'free at the point of delivery', and available to all was orthodox medicine. He describes the state-sponsored NHS as being dominated by 'the drug treatment and surgical interventions of orthodox medicine', thus relegating alternative therapies to the private health care market (Saks 1994: 86).

Orthodox medicine occupies a position of power and dominance over alternative medicine, as illustrated by the definitions of alternative practices offered by professional organisations such as the British Medical Association. The BMA draws a distinction between complementary therapies and alternative practices: the former are defined as treating patients while they are receiving drug therapy from a registered doctor, and the latter as treating patients *in place of* a registered doctor. The BMA offers a definition of orthodox medicine based principally on *who d*elivers the treatment, in this case a 'registered medical practitioner' (BMA 1993: 7). In a similar vein the definition of 'non-conventional' medicine centres around *what it is not*, that is orthodox, rather than considering *what it is* in terms of the concepts of health and disease underpinning alternative practices. Non-conventional medicine is defined as 'those forms of treatment which are not widely used by orthodox health care professions, and the skills of which are not taught as part of the undergraduate curriculum of orthodox medical and paramedical health care courses' (BMA 1993: 7). Saks (1994) argues that orthodox medicine has conducted a 'strong campaign' against its alternative competitors and draws on evidence from a report by the BMA published in 1986. This report, he suggests, 'extolled the scientific aspects of modern biomedicine, whilst at the same time generally depicting alternative medicine as superstitious dogma' (Saks 1994: 88). Supporters of orthodox medicine are keen to point out the importance of the patient having 'faith' in alternative practitioners and argue that this reinforces the message that the therapy will work. In contrast, it is suggested that orthodox medicine does not depend on this element of faith but on its proven ability to eradicate disease.

Question

Go back to the descriptions of homoeopathy and acupuncture. Can you recognise the concepts of health in the descriptions offered in Figure 4.1?

Alternative concepts of health

The following discussion requires you to draw on the examples of specific practices outlined above. The central elements of alternative medicine are detailed in Figure 4.1:

Alternative medicine	Biomedicine
Health as a balance of opposing forces within the body	Health as the absence of disease.
Disease understood as indicating the presence of negative, disruptive forces within the body. Symptoms are the product of the body's attempts to rid it of toxic substances.	Disease as defined in relation to a specific part of the body. Essentially, disease is understood as a deviation from normal functoning
'Reading' the body, examining dietary habits lifestyles and constitution types to achieve diagnosis	Diagnosis achieved by examining the form and structure of specific organisms and the degree to which the presence of a disease indicates a deviation from normal functioning
Therapy is based on an attempt to strengthen vitalising, positive forces within the body.	Therapy consists of attempts to destroy or suppress disease.

FIGURE 4.1   *Alternative medicine: concepts of health (Aakster 1993)*

Attempts to describe particular alternative practices and to detail what is specific about the concepts of health underpinning this approach reveal the essential differences between alternative medicine and the biomedical model. The discussion has sought to draw your attention to differing conceptions of health, disease and the relationship between mind, body and spirit. Biomedicine has sought to emphasise a further distinction between itself and alternative practices by asserting the supremacy of science over superstition. Previous discussions of biomedicine have dealt with its commitment to scientific methods free from social or political bias (BMA, cited in Saks 1992). The scientific observation of natural phenomena allows for the development of laws governing such phenomena and, perhaps most significantly, such laws and the resulting 'facts' can be said to be valid because the results can be reproduced repeatedly, proving their validity. This reproducibility of results, it is argued, cannot be matched by alternative medicine.

Links

See Chapter 3 for a detailed discussion of medicine as a dominant discourse.

The juxtaposition of 'scientific' medicine and 'unscientific' alternative practices leaves little scope for debate, as both sides appear to base their arguments on criteria not accepted by the other. It is biomedicine, however, that enjoys the dominant position as *the* established form of medicine. An essential element of this dominance can be traced back to a wide acceptance of the validity of science and scientific methods during **the Enlightenment**. The practice and philosophy of alternative medicine is, arguably, at a distinct disadvantage because science has reached the status of 'truth'. In the opening chapter, you were introduced to some of the basic elements of a post-modern critique of **society** and knowledge. Postmodernism is critical and sceptical of attempts to offer single, monolithic explanations of any phenomenon and so the whole basis of rational scientific knowledge has been questioned. Saks (1998: 204) argues that this critique of 'science, reason and enlightenment' provides a useful tool with which to reappraise the philosophical basis of alternative medical practices. Since post-modernism is characterised by 'the acceptance of multiple realities and coexisting narratives' (ibid.) it is possible to appraise the relative merits of alternative medicine and biomedicine in such a way that both are accepted as different but equally valid conceptions of the body, health and disease. Interestingly, the British Holistic Medical Association also draws attention to changes in modes of thinking and in particular to an acceptance of the non-scientific in terms of recognising the significance of human spirit and conscience. It argues that medicine in the twenty-first century will increasingly come to recognise the significance of the relationships between the mind, body and spirit and the human capacity to alter both the internal and the external environment (www.bhma.org).

Choosing to use alternative medicine

Alternative medicine clearly demonstrates the possibility of a philosophical challenge to the dominance of orthodox medicine. It should also be evident from the critique of medicine presented in the preceding chapter, that the practice of orthodox medicine is also ripe for criticism. Looking at the reasons for increasing use of alternative and complementary health care, McQuaide (2005) points to several trends in wider society. These indicate a growing individualism and dissociation from civic society and mainstream medicine. This ties in with Putnam's (2000) ideas on the decline of civic society in the US. Contemporary Americans are less likely to direct their efforts towards communal goals and activities and instead seek private solutions to their problems. Alternative health care fits this trend, as often the individual seeks out an alternative therapy for themselves as opposed to engaging with something like the NHS, with its communal orientation to health.

In relation to mainstream medicine, McQuaide makes the point that it is the unequal power relationship that puts people off using such services. More equal and participatory relationships are sought in alternative therapies and that appears to be one of their main attractions. Earlier work by Sharma (1992) found that in general people used alternative medicine because they placed a high value on what they found to be the more equal and informed relationship between practitioners and patients and because of the importance attached to the consideration of the personal circumstances of their illness. Further to this point, Coward (1993) argues that bio-medicine has not only medicalised many aspects of human existence but has done so in an inhumane way. The examples of iatrogenic practices discussed in Chapter 3 included a consideration of the harmful side-effects of drugs as well as examples of medical interventions, such as surgery, that have resulted in harm to the patient. The later discussion of mental health will also illustrate that the practice of medicine, as well as specific forms of treatment, has been uncaring and inhumane. The supposed neutrality of biomedicine, its ability to see disease as a purely biological entity, may not always be perceived as beneficial. As Coward comments, a purely rational expla-nation of disease as arbitrary does not, perhaps, satisfy a more fundamental need to understand why our own life has been affected in this way.

In addition to these individualistic currents, McQuaide also notes the influence of the baby boomer generation (those born between 1945 and 1960). As a generation they grew up with counter-cultural ideas strongly influenced by the 'hippie' idealism of the 1960s where nature and all things natural enjoyed a strong profile. Alternative health care, with its associations of being natural, neatly mirrors the culture that this generation were part of in their youth. This preference for all things natural, coupled with a desire to maintain health by purchasing that health care, has opened up a con-siderable market for alternative health care. This has to be tempered by acknowledg-ing that it is only really a viable option for those with a disposable income. Other reasons for the popularity of alternative medicine are identified in Figure 4.2.

We have highlighted the assumed advantages of alternative practices over orthodox medicine. However, these practices themselves have been subject to critical scrutiny. Commentators such as Coward have emphasised the individualistic assessment of health underpinning many alternative practices. Such an approach can be contrasted with the **social model of health** which draws our attention to the social, economic and cultural determinants of health. Chapter 6, examining class inequalities in health, seeks to place patterns of morbidity and mortality in a social context. There is wide-spread acceptance within the discipline of **sociology** that economic and social factors have a significant impact upon health outcomes. Sociologists of health do not deny the importance of **agency** (that is to say the capacity of individuals to act rather than be acted upon) but maintain that agency has its limitations. In contrast, Coward argues, alternative medicine stresses the extent to which individuals can determine their health status and an explanation that leads almost inevitably to the conclusion that individu-als are responsible for their own health regardless of their social circumstances.

- **The limits of biomedicine**
  Biomedicine is unable to 'cure' certain conditions.
  Biomedicine does not place enough emphasis on the causes of illness and is preoccupied with relieving symptoms.
  The side-effects of biomedical treatment are potentially harmful.
  Biomedical treatment is often too drastic and too invasive.

- **The benefits of alternative medicine**
  Provides an explanation of the causes of ill health and disease in the context of a person's individual lifestyle.
  Provides a more egalitarian relationship between patient and practitioner.
  Offers an alternative to 'high-tech' medicine.
  Treats the whole person.
  Encourages individuals to take greater responsibility for their health.

- **The use of alternative medicine as an expression of postmodern society**
  Expresses a greater desire for self-determination and choice.
  Challenges the cutural dominance of biomedicine.
  Reflects a more general trend for maintaining the body through the purchase of consumer goods and services.

FIGURE 4.2   *Explaining why people use alternative medicine (Sharma 1992; Coward 1993; Lupton 1995)*

Links

A detailed discussion of the regulated body is provided in Chapter 10.

This appeal to the individual is, Coward suggests, part of a cultural obsession with the performance and appearance of the body. It is important to note, however, that a central theme in the world of the 'worried well' is an obsession with appearance in terms of the body as a project, something owned by the individual and open to change and development by them. The widespread popularity, for example, of diets to lose weight, fitness to tone the body, and cosmetic surgery to alter it, are evidence of the new significance attached to the body. Working on the body to alter or enhance its appearance is represented as a matter of choice and self-determination. Good health and poor health, therefore, become matters of personal responsibility and, as Lupton reminds us, contain strong moral overtones of how we ought to care for the body.

Coward argues that part of the attraction of alternative medicine is its association with the natural world and the healing power of nature (cited in Lupton 1995: 126). Like the concept of 'science' with its association with the values of rationality, objectivity and progress, 'nature' is closely linked to ideas of virtue, goodness and purity (ibid. 127). Such an association suggests that nature and natural remedies are implicitly good for you and inevitably preferable to artificial substances such as pharmacological drugs. Lupton argues that it is impossible to support such a clear-cut distinction between natural and artificial substances since 'many naturally occurring substances can be toxic, and many chemicals are derived from naturally occurring substances' (ibid. 126). Many freely available herbal remedies carry the potential to be harmful when not taken in an appropriate manner. One such example, for the treatment of depression, would be the use of St John's wort, available over the counter and capable of being used even when a diagnosis of depression has not been made. It is perhaps ironic to note that, at a time when the use and efficacy of drugs are subject to more stringent regulation (through, for example, NHS Quality Improvement Scotland and the National Institute for Clinical Excellence in England and Wales) and when there is a requirement for pharmaceutical manufacturers to provide detailed patient information, natural remedies are not subject to the same degree of regulation. Most herbal remedies are in fact not classified as medicine and, therefore, are not subject to the same requirement for testing and regulation as artificial substances.

This chapter has described and analysed two challenges to the dominance of biomedicine by feminist critiques and by alternative medicine.

Conclusion

Following on from some points made earlier, we discussed here how medicine encroaches on many aspects of life that were traditionally outside its reach. Pregnancy and childbirth are good examples of this impulse of medicine not just to take control but also to redefine a natural state of being (in this case, for women) as being closer to illness than to health. Control is exercised in two ways: first by locating the place of delivery away from the home and into the hospital and therefore into medicine's 'home turf; second, less status and importance is attached to women's experiences and their interpretations of pregnancy and childbirth. This can be done overtly by overriding their concerns, or more subtly by framing pregnancy and childbirth as a time of risk and danger and thereby raising fears that the pregnancy is more likely to go wrong as opposed to right.

One should be careful not to see it all as 'one-way-traffic', where people meekly submit to medical control. The growth of alternative or complementary medicine provides an example where disenchantment with mainstream medicine is visible and where people make active choices to seek other forms of health care. Alternative medicine offers the promise of the individualistic and holistic care that is supposedly absent in mainstream medicine. It also reflects other processes apparent in late modernity, such as a focus on individualistic, as opposed to collective, solutions and a belief that natural remedies are superior to (and safer than) scientific or technological remedies. This may appear to be a more propitious state of affairs for people seeking a cure for an illness or to improve their health, but alternative medicine has one feature in common with its mainstream counterpart: there is little emphasis on the deeper structural or social aspects of health and illness. In the next section of this book we shall explore how structures (such as class, **ethnicity** and **gender**) are incredibly powerful in affecting and influencing health and illness.

SUMMARY POINTS

- The process of medicalisation has transformed natural experiences into medical ones. This is particularly true of pregnancy and childbirth.
- Medicine acts as a gatekeeper to reproductive technology. Decisions about access to reproductive technology are made not on the basis of medical and objective evidence but on the basis of prevailing social and cultural values.
- Authors such as Oakley argue that medicalisation has resulted in women patients being seen as passive recipients of care.
- Alternative medicine represents a fundamental challenge to the belief system underpinning biomedicine, as illustrated by two specific examples, homoeopathy and acupuncture.
- For an increasing number of people, alternative medicine represents a positive alternative to biomedicine.

Case study

Kathy was recently treated in hospital for a grade 'A' streptococcal infection that led to cellulitis, septicaemia and pneumonia. During her period of illness, she was given large doses of antibiotics and strong painkillers. The former placed a huge strain on her kidneys, while the latter made her drowsy and 'spaced out'.

Kathy never questioned the treatment she received even though she did not fully understand everything that she was told by the doctors and nurses.

Kathy is also a regular user of alternative medicine for the treatment of migraine. She has taken on board what she has been told by her homoeopathic practitioner and altered her diet and tried to deal positively with stressful situations.

1 How can Kathy be a user of orthodox medicine and alternative medicine?
2 For someone who has actively sought out a second opinion on her migraine and who has attempted to address the underlying causes of the condition through non-medical means, do you find it odd that she simply accepted what happened to her in hospital?
3 Talk to friends and colleagues and try and find out who uses or has used alternative medicine. Have they visited a practitioner or have they treated themselves by purchasing herbal medicines? For which conditions were people more likely to use alternative medicine?

Taking your studies further

This chapter will have helped you understand many of the key terms, concepts, theories and debates relating to medical dominance. Listed below are journal articles and books that will provide deeper and more detailed discussions of the points raised in this chapter. You will also find what is available on the companion website. This offers you downloads of relevant material, plus links to useful websites in addition to podcasts and other features.

Recommended reading

Books

Oakley, A. (2005) *The Ann Oakley Reader: Gender, Women and Social Science*. London: Policy Press.
Teijlingen E., van, Lowis, G., McCaffery, P. and Porter, M. (eds) (2004) *Midwifery and the Medicalization of Childbirth: Comparative Perspectives*, New York: Nova Science.
Turner, B.S., Tovey, P., Easthope, G. and Adams, J. (2003) *Mainstreaming Complementary and Alternative Medicine: Studies in Social Context*. London: Routledge.

Journal articles

Jackson, S. and Graham Scambler, G. (2007) 'Perceptions of evidence-based medicine: traditional acupuncturists in the UK and resistance to biomedical modes of evaluation', *Sociology of Health and Illness*, 29 (3): 412–29.

McQuaide, M.M. (2005) 'The rise of alternative health care: a sociological account', *Social Theory and Health*, 3 (4): 286–301.

On the companion website

Stevenson, F. (2004) 'Images of nature in relation to mood modifying medicines: a user perspective', *Health*, 8 (4): 241–62.

5

Evidence and enquiry: an overview of sociological research

MAIN POINTS

- Research is integral to sociology, as it both provides evidence for existing claims about society and also prompts new ways of thinking and theorising about society.
- Research is a practical activity, which needs careful planning and coordination to realise its aims.
- There are two main methodological traditions: quantitative and qualitative.
- Quantitative methods focus mainly on statistical relationships, as gathered through surveys.
- Qualitative methods focus mainly on experiences, as gathered through interviews or focus groups.
- Research has to be ethically sound in order to prevent distress or harm for the people who participate in the research.

KEY CONCEPTS

Research, methods, quantitative, qualitative, interviews, surveys, ethnography, ethics.

Introduction

Research is integral to **sociology** and it is vital for the following two reasons. First, without research many of the insights and observations that sociologists put forward about **society** would have no validity or evidence to support the claim being made. So, for example, sociologists make claims that health is distributed unevenly across society, according to **class**, **gender** and **ethnicity**. If you turn to the various chapters on those social structures in Section 2, then you will find summaries of some of the evidence that sociologists use to give credence to those statements. Second, research makes sociologists think about society in new ways, with the result either of challenging existing ways of thinking about something or raising questions that have never been posed before. A useful example here is Bury's work on chronic illness. Following his interviews with young people with rheumatoid arthritis, Bury drew attention to the social aspects of chronic illness. His research helped to generate the concept of 'disrupted biography', which enables sociologists to gain insights and explain the challenges that chronic illness can present to people with conditions such as multiple sclerosis or Parkinson's disease.

In this chapter, we will be exploring some of the main issues concerning the focus of sociological research and the various methods that are involved in trying to find out about society. We will begin by considering whether or not sociology is a science, before moving on to some of the nuts and bolts of going about developing a research project. Attention will then turn to reflecting on types of research methods and how they reveal different aspects of society and how people experience society. Finally, a review of ethical issues will examine why it is important to provide safeguards for the people who participate in a research project and some of the steps necessary to do so.

5.1 Sociology as a science

As discussed in Chapter 1, sociology shares many of the characteristics of other sciences. These characteristics include using rigorous and systematic methods during research and developing from that research logical and theoretically informed discussions and conclusions. To that extent sociology is a science, but it does have one quite notable difference in contrast to the natural sciences. That difference is in what sociologists study. Sociologists have as their object of study *people* in a *society*. Studying people is quite different from, let us say, looking at how two different chemicals combine in a test tube. Chemicals are not aware of themselves, nor are they capable of acting on their own volition and making their own decisions. People, on the contrary, are self-aware, conscious, and can make up their own minds and purposefully act accordingly. Therefore, we have to be alert not just to recording and observing what transpires when people interact and engage in activities but also *why* they interact and the motives and thinking behind their engagement with certain activities. So, for example, in Chapter 4 we shall look at the increasing uptake of alternative therapies. Much of the research in that area explores why people are opting for such therapies and the motives and reasons that lie behind their actions. What it reveals is that many people opt for alternative therapies because of disillusionment with mainstream medicine and a desire to be treated in an individual and holistic manner.

Links

See Chapter 1 for more information on sociology as science.

5.2 Doing research

Engaging in research requires a great deal of planning and prior thought. Getting the planning right (or as right as possible) before any actual fieldwork is carried out can make a decisive difference to the success of the final project. There is a great deal to organise and think about. Building the research project on a firm foundation is essential if the research is to be able to answer the questions that it sets out to examine. Research is very much a practical activity shaped by a variety of constraints and considerations, where the researcher has to be aware of and attuned to what they can deliver rather than what they might wish to do. Let us now look at what the planning stage involves.

Research question

First of all, it is crucial to work out what the **research question** is, and to be absolutely clear about what the research is trying to find out. A research question is what the research seeks to do, and what aspects of the social world need to be understood. What initially prompts a research question is quite varied. Sometimes the research question is posed by theoretical concerns to prove or disprove an existing **theory**, sometimes by a knowledge gap that is noted in the literature or sometimes

Research question refers to the aspect of the social world that is to be investigated. **Literature review** refers to a systematic analysis of all published material that is of interest or relevant to the research. **Method** refers to the way in which the actual data is gathered. **Analysis** means making sense of the data and deriving conclusions that inform the research question. **Dissemination** refers to making the results and conclusions of the research known to a wider audience.

because a funding body (for example a local authority or a charity) needs information on some aspect of its service.

Once the research question has been formulated, you have to be aware of the practical limitations of what you are seeking to do. Research is very much the 'art of the possible' – understanding what resources one has to put into play and how much time is available to do it. A potential trap in all research is that the initial ambition of a research project is too big and to realise the aims would require excessive amounts of time, funding and people. Often, planning research involves honing the research question down to a very tight set of aims that can actually be answered and can be practically pursued.

So, for example, you might wish to research how having a chronic illness has impacted on all of the sufferers' sense of self, changed the dynamics of family and personal relationships and so on. This would involve perhaps interviewing everyone in the UK about what differences and experiences they have encountered in their lives since the onset of, let us say, multiple sclerosis, HIV/AIDS, or Parkinson's disease. Undoubtedly, if this could be done, it would be a very valuable piece of research; however, given the numbers of people to be interviewed (potentially tens of thousands), the time (months, if not years) needed to do it and the army of research assistants and interviewers necessary to carry out the interviews, plus the no doubt astronomical cost, then it simply could not happen. Instead, it would be much more practical to select just one chronic illness, for example multiple sclerosis (MS). Again, one would not be able to interview everyone with MS, for the same reasons as before, given the numbers of people with the condition and the time and financial implications. This in turn means reducing the intended number of people that could be asked to participate in the research. The main point is that one always has to be practical in what can be achieved and to make sure that the research question can be addressed in a relevant and meaningful way.

Literature review

The next stage involves going through the literature that already exists on the subject. It is highly unlikely that any piece of research is entirely novel or unique. A great deal (if not all!) of research follows on from and is informed by other pieces of research. It is therefore essential to consult and read all the other existing relevant material. Doing so will aid the researcher in many ways. It will provide an awareness of the main findings and issues that have been put forward so far and how new research can contribute to this body of knowledge. Sometimes this contribution will illuminate gaps in the previous research or offer different or critical counterpoints to what other researchers have found and discussed.

Choosing an appropriate research method

Once the research question has been posed and the literature reviewed, attention turns to how to actually do the research. This requires the selection of an appropriate **method** to answer the research question. In some respects, this will involve choosing between quantitative and qualitative methods. The differences between the two approaches will be explored in section 5.3, but essentially quantitative methods tells us about 'how many' and 'how much', while the qualitative methods answer questions of 'what', 'how' and 'why' (Green and Thorogood 2004: 5).

Analysing the data

Data unfortunately does not 'speak' for itself and requires further work, to produce meaningful information. The actual type of data that is collected determines the type of analysis that is required. For statistical data one of the most common approaches is to use some form of software package, such as SPSS. This allows the researcher to model any relationships and variables that the research set out to find. Qualitative data, on the other hand, requires a different approach, it is the spoken words of the research participants. This has to be fully transcribed (typed out) before themes can be identified in the various participants' responses.

Disseminating research findings

Gathering, analysing and interpreting data and reaching a conclusion or raising important issues as a result of research is not the end of the process. Of equal importance is what one does with the research when it is complete and how results are conveyed to the wider world. In terms of reaching a wider audience, Burawoy (2004) has made an appeal for what he terms 'public sociology', arguing that sociologists should strive to make their research and ideas relevant and understandable to the wider society. It is not only academics who are interested in what research has to say; other people, such as user groups, those involved in the study or policy makers and, indeed, the public at large are also concerned.

5.3 Quantitative and qualitative methods

As outlined above, it is important to select the correct method that is going to help you answer your research question. Within sociological research it can be useful to distinguish between two different broad methodological approaches. These are

Quantitative research refers to mainly statistically-based research that is useful for answering research questions that focus on measuring the extent and range of particular phenomena.

Qualitative research refers mainly to interview-based research that seeks to find out the meanings that people attach to their experiences and actions.

quantitative and **qualitative research** methods. Each method has its own orientation to the ways in which we can investigate society. On a very simple level quantitative research methods place an emphasis on statistics and measuring the differences, relationships and extent of various social phenomena, while qualitative research methods place an emphasis on how people experience and make sense of the society in which they live.

We shall look at specific examples of qualitative methods shortly, but first it is useful to look at some of the debates that have surrounded both approaches as they can help us to understand their relative advantages and disadvantages.

Much of the debate over the years concerning methods has centred on which approach is the more 'effective' and the more 'scientific'. Qualitative research has often been criticised for being unscientific in that it is closer to a form of journalism, given its emphasis on interviews as opposed to, for example, the randomised control sampling and statistical techniques prevalent in certain quantitative research. Other criticisms are that qualitative researchers lack the impartiality and the objectivity that is supposedly part of quantitative research.

Quantitative research, on the other hand, has been taken to task on many grounds. Even though quantitative methods can tell us a great deal of useful information and are ideal for establishing predictive information, various problems and drawbacks have been identified. For example, much of the survey work on class and health inequalities clearly indicates that one can predict that people found in the lower social classes will have a greater chance of increased morbidity and early mortality. While this is very valuable, this form of research only tells us about one level of social reality. What is missings are insights into how people experience and construct their worlds. The reliance that quantitative methods have on statistical modelling can also be problematic. In compiling and cross-referencing statistics some of the important features of the social world are lost, such as context and the power relationships between people.

Even though there are strong arguments for and against both methods, they should be thought of as complementary. It is the strengths of each that should be appreciated and those strengths in turn should be matched with the research question in hand. So, for example, if the purpose of the research is to investigate the frequency of consultations on a certain condition (for example, depression) by social class in a certain area, then a quantitative method, such as a survey, would be useful. If, on the other hand, the research seeks to explore what it means to be a working-class person with depression then a qualitative method, such as an in-depth interview, would be the preferred option.

The discussion above has presented the choice of quantitative and qualitative methods as being an either/or option, where one has to be selected rather than the other. Increasingly, we are seeing the use of mixed methods, where both methods are used in the same piece of research.

Quantitative method: Surveys

If a very large population is to be researched then a survey can be a useful way to do this. Surveys can take a variety of forms. Traditionally, they have involved the distribution of postal questionnaires or the conducting of structured interviews (either in person or by telephone); though with current technology surveys can be completed using websites or other online media. A defining characteristic of the survey approach is the way in which questions are asked. Questions are tightly *structured*, involving a specific set of questions, asked in a designated order, usually with a limited range of answers. The purpose of such a fixed set of questions and answers is to allow information to be collated and compared across a distinct population. Variables (for example, age, class, ethnicity and gender) can therefore be identified and various associations can be made.

Examples of survey questions

(3) Please circle which of the following responses is closest to what you thought overall of the Middlefield Wellman Project.

Very satisfied   Satisfied   Happy   Dissatisfied   Very dissatisfied

(4) How often did you attend the Middlefield Wellman Project? Circle as appropriate.

On one occasion   Two or three occasions   On four or more occasions

Qualitative method: Interviews

One very common research approach in the sociology of health and illness is the in-depth interview. Typically, this is carried out on a one-to-one basis where highly detailed information and data are elicited by talking with someone who meets the criteria of the research project. Most interviews last between one and two hours and are usually recorded using a tape or digital recorder. This recording is then transcribed so that the interview can be analysed.

In many respects, one can think of an interview as a purposeful conversation where the actual data collected is in the form of what someone says (Green and Thorogood 2004). It is up to the interviewer to guide or facilitate the conversation. This can be done in two ways. There is a *structured* approach (as in the survey approach outlined above) but more commonly in interviews one follows a *semi-structured* approach. This is very much a 'looser' and more open technique. The interviewer will have certain topics she will wish to explore with the emphasis being on allowing the interviewees to express and communicate what they feel or have experienced about what is being researched. So, instead of having a fixed agenda of questions the interviewer will have an outline of areas or issues to be addressed and will raise those areas or issues as and when is appropriate during the interview. This can mean being flexible and not rigidly adhering to a pre-set order or question format or style.

Conducting a semi-structured interview requires certain skills, techniques and styles of approaches. One should remember that someone is giving up their time to discuss what can be quite intimate and personal details of their life, and due respect should be accorded. It also entails behaving and acting in certain ways before, during and after the interview. Before the interview takes place it is important to identify and create a non-threatening and relaxed atmosphere for the interviewee. This can involve identifying a venue that is familiar to the person who is being interviewed: this could include many different places, such as their home or place of work, so long as they are comfortable there. During the interview the interviewer should be attentive to what the interviewee is discussing and always appear interested. This can be achieved in a variety of ways. Often, quite subtle actions such as nodding one's head or briefly commenting on how useful or important something is that the interviewee has said are the most effective. Engaging with someone in this way also makes it more likely that the interview will elicit the information that the research requires. Questions should always be open (that is, not questions that have yes or no responses) and allow the interviewee room to explore issues they regard as being important.

Examples of semi-structured questions

How did you feel about having physiotherapists and occupational therapists coming into your home?

Could you tell me more about what you felt when you heard the diagnosis from the specialist?

Importantly, the interview is not about obtaining some form of universal 'truth' nor should it necessarily match an 'objective reality'. This is one possible objection to the interview approach: that it may not be able to gather accurate data, and therefore any conclusions reached may be invalid. This could be because the inter-viewee is unable to recall specific events, or has a particular view (or bias) about the research topic. However, it is how the person sees *their* world that is what is being sought in an interview and not whether or not it matches some other view of the world (for example the researcher's or the views of a powerful social group, such as the medical profession).

Focus groups

Another highly popular method is the focus group approach. This involves a small interactive group of people discussing and commenting on issues and questions prompted by the researcher. As with interviews, a focus group will also be recorded and then transcribed for subsequent analysis and, as with in-depth inter-views, the group can last anywhere between one and two hours. Who actually populates the focus group is dependent on the research questions and aims. Sometimes this can be a wide range of people if the researcher wishes to explore how take-up and perception of, let us say, alternative therapies differs by social class. Other times it can be people who share a particular characteristic, for example depression, if the research is investigating the day-to-day experiences of people with mental health problems.

Focus groups can be very useful research tools in a number of ways. Firstly, unlike interviews, where there is a one-to-one conversation between the interviewer and the interviewee, talking with a group of people is much closer to how people interact in the rest of their lives and therefore creates a more 'natural' and 'common-place' environment, hopefully making it easier for people to contribute what they want. For the researcher this natural aspect of the focus group also allows insights into group dynamics and the ways in which people express their ideas and relate to others. Secondly, the views and experiences of a number of people can be accessed in a relatively short period of time. Given the time and financial considerations that affect most research, this can be a very appealing option.

There can be some problems with focus groups and those problems relate to the very fact that it is a group. As in any social situation, where a group of people are gathered together to discuss a particular subject, some people will be more vocal than others, while some people may feel too nervous to contribute. It can be diffi-cult to keep everyone on track and the setting of ground rules, such as asking group members not to interrupt someone who is making a contribution, are usually nec-essary. The points made about successful interviewing also apply here in that the interviewer needs to be attentive and interested throughout, while creating a relaxed and participative atmosphere.

Ethnography and participant observation

Wogan (2004) playfully refers to ethnography as 'deep hanging out'. This remark is not as flippant as it sounds, since ethnography is about spending a great deal of time with a group of people in order to discover how they see the world, while observing, sharing and participating in their everyday experiences. Sometimes this can involve just witnessing what is going on or perhaps (though this can be problematic) going 'undercover' and attempting to become one of the group which is being studied.

One of the most well known examples of ethnography in sociology is Goffman's *Asylums* (1961). In this study, Goffman adopted the role of an assistant to the athletic director (similar to what we would call a physiotherapist today) and spent as much time as possible talking to and interacting with patients in St Elizabeth's, a hospital for people with mental illnesses. The aim of the research was to investigate the effects that institutional life had on the identities and experiences of those patients. Famously, he identified the processes that lead to institutionalisation, a state of being where an individual's own identity is replaced by an identity that suits the requirements of an institution. Reflecting on the usefulness of ethnography after he had completed the research Goffman noted:

> It was then and still is my belief that any group of persons – prisoners, primitives, pilots or patients – develop a life of their own that becomes meaningful, reasonable, and normal once you get close to it, and that a good way to learn about any of those worlds is to submit oneself in the company of the members to the daily round of petty contingencies to which they are subject. (Goffman 1961: 8)

What Goffman is putting forward here is that only by being with a group of people for a length of time can one come close to understanding the contours and rhythms of their lives. This is unlike the other methods that were discussed above, as they only capture a snapshot – albeit what can be a fairly detailed snapshot – of the lives and experiences of certain groups of people. Ethnography can help to get into the nitty-gritty of social life and reveal how people construct and produce their day-to-day lives.

One issue that all researchers face before embarking on ethnographic research is how much information to divulge about themselves to the group or **community** they are going to be studying. This is an issue because there are two approaches that one can adopt during an ethnographic research: covert or overt. A covert approach entails a certain level of concealment and deception. This could mean pretending that you are one of the group or someone who would normally be associated with the group. For some research projects this may be entirely appropriate, but can be challenging for a number of reasons. Let us take a slightly exaggerated example to illustrate what a covert ethnography might entail. If one was to do an ethnographic study of the stresses and strains facing junior doctors one could pretend to be a junior doctor. This would allow the researcher first-hand observations of the actual experiences of junior doctors as they work through their various shifts. One would be able to witness the rhythms and contours of what causes the most stress and the various coping strategies junior doctors may employ. On one level this would appear to be an excellent method of gathering some very detailed and accurate information. There are, however, certain drawbacks associated with this covert approach: most importantly, would the researcher have the necessary skills to pass himself off as a doctor? This is highly unlikely, given the number of years required to amass such specialised knowledge and most sociologists simply would not have time to do that. There are also ethical issues (more of which in section 5.4). If you were pretending to be a junior doctor then this would inevitably require the treating of patients, which is where such an approach would run into severe problems, as it would be utterly irresponsible to do this.

An overt approach, on the other hand, requires the researcher to disclose their identity as a researcher and be up-front as to what they are doing. This may avoid some of the ethical issues outlined above but it can lead to other problems, the main one being that the naturalistic flow of events is disrupted. Having someone observing (or 'hanging out') and recording what is happening is highly unusual and this can make people reflect on what they are doing and interact in uncharacteristic ways.

An important feature of ethnography is to keep a detailed account of what one observes and encounters. As Crang and Cook (2007) point out, keeping a thorough detailed notebook (though this could include all sorts of digital media) is an essential part of the ethnography. It is where observations, thoughts and conversations are recorded for future analysis. In effect, the notebook *is* the data and what is recorded in the notebook becomes the basis for the conclusions or conjectures that are advanced from the research.

Analysing qualitative data

As we discussed earlier, one of the defining attributes of qualitative research is the collection of the spoken word during an interview or focus group. This forms the data of the research. Analysing such data requires a distinctive approach in that the researcher is not applying mathematical formulae or models to the data, as is usual with quantitative data. Rather, one of the most common approaches is for the researcher is to identify themes within the data. This involves going through the transcripts from the interviews and 'coding' what is said. Unlike slotting numbers into a software package or into neat equations this is not always a 'neat' task. It often means scribbling notes and annotations on transcripts, cutting up those transcripts or attaching stick-on notes and keeping memos. Crang and Cook (2007: 133) capture this part of the research project well, when they say:

> It is a process that involves doing nitty-gritty things with paper, pens, scissors, computers and software. It's about chopping up, (re)ordering, (re)contextualising and (re)assembling the data we have so diligently constructed. It's about translating a messy process into a neat product.

Let us now turn more closely to this 'messy process'. If we follow what is referred to as a 'grounded theory' approach (one of the most commonly used in health research) we begin with what Strauss (1987) calls 'open coding'. Here the researcher reads though the transcript and begins to note down what she or he deems to be significant, important or something that crops up several times in the transcript. There is a certain amount of trial-and-error' in doing this. Some codes will work and emerge throughout the transcripts while others will not. The codes one attaches could be codes that the researcher sees emerging in the transcripts or can be *in vivo* codes: these are the ways that the participants involved in the research see the world in which they live and think about their own experiences. There is a cyclical process at play here, with the researcher going back through the transcripts continually refining and 'neatening up' the codes that have been previously identified. This cyclical process stops either when no new concepts emerge out of the data or when the existing concepts cannot be refined any further.

Once no new codes can be generated or further honed from existing codes the next stage involves trying to make sense of all the different codes and seeking out ways of making them meaningful by looking for connections and relationships. This is referred to as *axial coding*.

After all the relationships have been worked out and identified, attention can turn to the final stage. This is where you try to work out what the one central or *core category* that helps to explain what all the other codes and themes means. Essentially, this entails taking an overview of those codes and themes and seeing what commonality runs through all of them. This may involve a more theoretical or abstract code than the other themes that have been discussed so far.

In the example given in Table 5.1, we can see how this might take place. This is a transcript of research on the psycho-social health of workers in a Scottish call centre. The research sought to investigate the link between how the requirements of performing emotional labour all day to people down a telephone line created certain emotional states that in turn had possible health consequences.

Ethics refers to guiding principles and considerations concerning the conduct of the researcher in ensuring that no harm is done to the physical and emotional well-being of those who participate in the research.

5.4 Ethics

Invariably, with research into health, sociologists encounter ethical issues; especially when the research is investigating issues that are quite personal and intimate for

TABLE 5.1 *Example of coding themes on a transcript of an interview*

Line	Interview	Themes
101	**Int:** So, what really gets you down at work?	
102	**Steve**: Gets me down? Aye, heaps of things!	
103	Mainly, it's that they're always looking at you,	**Surveillance**
104	you know, always got their nose in what you're	
105	doing. It's like, you know, they dinnae trust you.	**Trust**
106	Hate that!	**Anger**
107	**Int:** Anything else?	
108	**Steve:** As I said – heaps! The other thing is that	
109	you are not allowed to make your own	**Lack of autonomy**
110	decisions. If it does not fit their perceived little	
111	wee plans, then ye cannae just go ahead and do	
112	it. Everything is controlled, and worked out to	
113	so minute a degree. And you've got to stick to it,	
114	even if it doesnae work or takes longer, know	
115	what I mean? They just don't trust you with	**Trust**
116	anything!	
117	**Int:** How does that make you feel?	
118	**Steve:** Well, angry again, but pretty depressed as	**Anger/depression**
119	well. It's all day with your heid against the	
120	same brick wall.	**Lack of job fulfilment**

the subjects of the study, or potentially involves accessing confidential medical and clinical information. Sociologists often have to seek ethical approval for their research due to the very real possibility of causing either distress or upset. This can include, for example, unintentionally making information public concerning diagnosis of chronic illness, revealing someone's sexuality or their views on other people in a user group. All of this could cause embarrassment but could also seriously damage and hinder relationships or future courses of treatment and care for the subject.

To avoid causing problems, the researcher is required to follow two courses of action. The first is to adhere to a code of **ethics**. In the UK all sociologists should consult and follow the British Sociological Association's (BSA) code of ethics, which outlines the considerations that sociologists should follow when engaging in research activity. Part of the guidelines, on relationships with participants in this instance, are shown below. A neat summary of the code, as well as good all-round advice when engaging in research with people, is 'to do no harm'.

Examples of ethics codes

The Economics, Social and Research Council:
http://www.esrc.ac.uk/ESRCInfoCentre/Images/ESRC_Re_Ethics_Frame_
tcm6-11291.pdf
The College of Occupational Therapists:
http://www.cot.org.uk/members/publications/ethics/pdf/code0605.pdf
The Chartered Society of Physiotherapy.
http://www.csp.org.uk/uploads/documents/csp_effecprac_res07.pdf

Relationships with research participants

- Sociologists have a responsibility to ensure that the physical, social and psychological well-being of research participants is not adversely affected by the research. They should strive to protect the rights of those they study, their interests, sensitivities and privacy, while recognising the difficulty of balancing potentially conflicting interests.
- Because sociologists study the relatively powerless as well as those more powerful than themselves, research relationships are frequently characterised by disparities of power and status. Despite this, research relationships should be characterised, whenever possible, by trust and integrity.
- In some cases, where the public interest dictates otherwise and particularly where power is being abused, obligations of trust and protection may weigh less heavily. Nevertheless, these obligations should not be discarded lightly.
- As far as possible participation in sociological research should be based on the freely given informed consent of those studied. This implies a responsibility on the sociologist to explain in appropriate detail, and in terms meaningful to participants, what the research is about, who is undertaking and financing it, why it is being undertaken, and how it is to be disseminated and used.
- Research participants should be made aware of their right to refuse participation whenever and for whatever reason they wish.
  http://www.britsoc.co.uk/equality/ 63.htm

Many other bodies have their own ethical codes and they too are worth consulting. Overall, these ethical codes share similar concerns about maintaining professional standards in terms of behaviour and not exposing participants in research to any harm or distress.

The second course of action involves submitting a proposal to an ethics committee. This could be an internal body, such as a university ethics committee, or an external body, such as the local NHS ethics committee. Due to heightened – and very real – concerns about people's rights, these have become increasingly common and, in some ways, increasingly demanding. In the proposal the researcher will outline what the study is about, what the possible risks to the people involved in the subject are, and what measures will be taken to avoid creating or encountering ethical problems. This can be quite complex and the ethical considerations and safeguards of the NHS in particular can be very demanding and thorough. Once clearance has been obtained from the committee, or the researcher has acted on their recommendations to enhance the protection of the people in the study, then the research can go ahead.

One very common ethical consideration, and something of vital importance when involving people in research, is that the researcher must obtain informed consent from those taking part in the research. This will involve providing them with an outline of what the research is about, what they will be asked to do in the research and how the information they provide will be handled, stored, and disseminated. Consent is usually sought by asking those who are taking part to sign a form that lays out the points just made. It is vital that at all times communication is in a way that is understandable to the respondent. When the research involves people who may not be able to understand what is being required of them, such as children, then some form of proxy consent is required.

Conclusion

Research is an essential part of the sociological project and provides both questions and answers in our attempts to understand society. The focus of sociological research though differs from that of the natural sciences. Sociologists are faced with the dynamic flow of an ever changing world animated by the actions of thinking and purposeful human beings. Understanding their motives, interpretations and experiences therefore forms a great deal of what sociologists do. This in turn affects and influences the research methods that are used in the pursuit of knowledge. In addition to the statistical profiles of the more familiar quantitative approaches, sociologists employ qualitative approaches, which seek to access and bring forward the motives and narratives of people in everyday life.

SUMMARY POINTS

- Research is a vital part of sociology.
- Sociological research is scientific like the natural sciences, but deals with purposeful self-aware people as opposed to inanimate objects.

- Research is a very practical activity and requires the researcher to be realistic in what they can do in order to meet their research question.
- Quantitative methods include surveys and mass questionnaires and are useful for establishing the size and extent of particular social phenomena.
- Qualitative methods include focus groups, in-depth interviews and ethnography and are useful for understanding the experiences and motives of people.
- Interviewing people requires certain skills so as to create an environment in which research participants feel at ease, where they can discuss and comment on their experiences.
- Ethical considerations are an important aspect of research. Care must be taken not to physically, psychologically or emotionally harm people who participate in the research.

Case study

The following tasks could be useful for you to consider in relation to the points raised above. Read the tasks and then reflect on the questions below

Task 1

Students are often young people who, when they move away from home for the first time, have to adapt quickly to being independent. Often universities find that first year is very stressful for students. As is discussed in this book, stress can be a cause of ill health. How would you research the issues that students face at this stage in their college and university careers and the effects this has on their health?

Task 2

Most universities have a range of students on a variety of courses. Intuitively one would think that students on health-related courses would have better or wider knowledge of health and have a more healthy lifestyle than students on non-health- related courses. How would you research this comparison between different cohorts of students?

Think about the following:

What would a suitable research question be?
Where would you look for previous literature on student experiences away from home?
What method would you use – quantitative or qualitative?
What problems may you encounter in doing the research?
What ethical issues would you have to be aware of? What permissions and consents would have to be obtained?

Taking your studies further

This chapter will have helped you understand many of the key terms, concepts, theories and debates relating to Sociological research. Listed below are journal articles and books that will provide deeper and more detailed discussions of the points raised in this chapter. You will also find what is available on the companion website. This offers downloads of relevant material, plus links to useful websites in addition to podcasts and other features.

Recommended reading

Bryman, A. (2001) *Social Research Methods*. Oxford: Oxford University Press.

Crang, M. and Cook, I. (2007) *Doing Ethnographies*. London: Sage.

Green, J. and Thorogood, N. (2004) *Qualitative Methods for Health Research*. London: Sage.

Hugman, R. (2005) *New Approaches in Ethics for the Caring Professions*. London: Palgrave MacMillan.

Mason, J. (2002) *Qualitative Researching*. London: Sage.

Richards, L. (2005) *Handling Qualitative Data: A Practical Guide*. London: Sage.

Seale, C. (1999) *The Quality of Qualitative Research*. London: Sage.

Silverman, D. (2001) *Interpreting Qualitative Data, 2nd edn*. London: Sage.

Strauss, A. L. and Corbin, J. (eds) (1997) *Grounded Theory in Practice*. Thousand Oaks, CA: Sage.

Strauss, A. L. and Corbin, J. (1998) *Basics of Qualitative Research: Techniques and Procedures for Developing Grounded Theory*. Thousand Oaks, CA: Sage.

On the companion website

You will find a selection of research-based articles that provide examples of the various research methods outlined in this chapter.

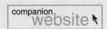

SECTION 2

Key Themes

6

Class and health

MAIN POINTS

- There are enduring differences between social classes in relation to health.
- In terms of early mortality, morbidity and a range of other health indicators disadvantaged groups have considerably poorer outcomes than advantaged groups.
- Substantial relative poverty is prevalent in the UK, with high levels of child poverty in many areas.
- Two current, and in many ways rival, theories attempt to explain class and health inequalities: the psycho-social and the neo-material.
- The psycho-social perspective highlights how societies lacking in social cohesion have poor health, while the neo-material perspective emphasises access to resources.

KEY CONCEPTS

Class, inequality, poverty, psycho-social explanations, neo-material explanations, place.

Introduction

If you are from a manual, or working-class, background you are, generally speaking, likely to die younger (see Figure 6.1), age faster and encounter more long-term limiting illnesses than someone from a non-manual, or middle-class, background. This lamentable state of affairs has been apparent in much of the research looking at **class** and health for some time now. Going back to the mid-1800s, Marx's collaborator Engels wrote about the poor health of the working classes in Manchester. He claimed that the levels of disease, illness and death were a form of 'social murder' committed by the bourgeoisie. More recently, landmark reports such as the Black Report published in 1980 and the Acheson Report published in 1998 both strongly indicated that which class you are in affects your health. A welter of other pieces of research further support that view. The problem for **sociology** though, is trying to explain just how class affects health.

This chapter will focus on class and health and, in doing so, will look at a variety of connected issues. We shall begin by exploring what we mean by class and some of the sociological theories of class. Attention will then turn to the extent of social inequalities in contemporary society, picking up on differences in such areas as wealth, income, poverty and education. Next will come a breakdown of the research and data on the extent of class and health inequalities.

6.1 What is class?

Class refers to a complex stratification of society based on access to and control of power, status and economic resources.

British readers of this book may have a certain idea of what class is: titled wealthy individuals in top hats on the one hand, and tracksuit-wearing 'hoodies' on the other hand. There may be something in these cultural differences in people's appearance; however, class is a complex and dynamic power relationship between people. Class societies are also distinct from other societies that are also stratified. For example, in feudal society distinctions between people were rigid, immobile and seen to be religiously ordained. The reason why you were a lord or a peasant was because God willed it that way and there was no way to change it. In contemporary capitalist societies one can be more socially mobile between classes. This is because, in many ways, you *achieve* your class position and it is not fixed by your birth. Though having said that, most people tend to stay in or near the class they were born into.

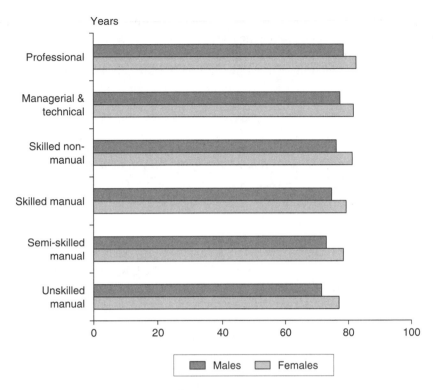

FIGURE 6.1   *Life expectancy by class and gender (ONS 2004: 6)*
Source: National Statistics website: www.statistics.gov.uk
Crown copyright material is reproduced with the permission of the Controller of HMSO
Reproduced under the terms of the Click-Use Licence

Class is, as mentioned before, more than just how people dress and speak. In fact, those forms of distinction are becomingly increasingly eroded in contemporary society. No longer do all workers in the City of London wear bowler hats, for instance. More importantly, it is the very real and dramatic differences between people, both economically and in terms of power, we must be aware of. It is those differences that lead to class differences. In section 3 of this chapter, we look at economic differences between classes. What we will see there is that considerable wealth is owned by a very small percentage while a sizeable percentage live on or near the poverty line. In terms of power, people in the higher social class have greater control over a whole range of resources. So for example, people in higher social classes generally have more control over how they organise their work, with less intervention from supervisors and managers. Indeed, they may be managers, meaning that they can control the working conditions of others. Also, by having greater income people in higher social classes will have greater control and power over their day-to-day lives: being able to afford foreign travel, eat organic food, or have more frequent leisure time, for example.

Question

Do you think class still exists today? If so, who do you think occupies the top of society and why?

Measuring class

Defining and measuring class can be very difficult. In the UK, official statistics up until 2001 used the Registrar-General's Social Class scheme (RGSC), a system that has been used since 1911. This was a descriptive, not a theoretical, approach that ranked six classes in order of what was commonly held to be occupational advantage. In 2001 the RGSC was replaced by the National Statistics Socio-economic Classification (NS-SEC). It is hoped that the new approach more accurately reflects current perceptions of both occupations and occupational advantage. This book was written at a time when official statistics changed from the one method to the other. You will see both in approaches used in this chapter and others. What the titles and numbers mean are laid out below (see Tables 6.1 and 6.2), and this should make it easier to read the various tables and graphs included here. It is, however, worth pointing out that both approaches have their good and bad points, but both provide much useful information.

Question

Which of the two ways of trying to classify class do you find the more convincing? Where do you think you would be classified as a student? Where do you think you will be classified when you graduate?

6.2 Health inequalities

We will now look a little more closely at the shape and extent of class and health inequalities. In the introduction we noted, and saw in Figure 6.1, that there was a great

TABLE 6.1   *Eight-class grouping of the National Statistics Socio-economic Classification*

Classification title	Examples of occupation
1 Higher managerial and professional occupations	Doctors, lawyers, dentists, professors, professional engineers
2 Lower managerial and professional occupations	School teachers, nurses, journalists, actors, police sergeants
3 Intermediate occupations	Airline cabin crew, secretaries
4 Small employers and own account workers	Non-professionals with fewer than 25 employees e.g.: self-employed builders, hairdressers or fishermen, shopkeepers with own shop
5 Lower supervisory and technical occupations	Train drivers, employed plumbers or electricians, foremen, supervisors
6 Semi-routine occupations	Shop assistants, postmen, security guards, call centre workers, care assistants
7 Routine occupations	Bus drivers, waitresses, cleaners, car park attendants, refuse collectors
8 Never worked and long-termed unemployed	People who have either never worked or are long-term unemployed and therefore cannot be classified

Source: National statistics website: www.statistics.gov.uk
Crown copyright material is reproduced with the permission of the Controller of HMSO
Reproduced under the terms of the Click-Use Licence

TABLE 6.2   *Registrar General's Social Class*

Non-manual		Examples of occupation
I	Professional	Doctors, lawyers, chartered accountants, professionally qualified engineers
II	Intermediate	Managers, school teachers, journalists
IIIN	Skilled non-manual	Clerks, cashiers, retail staff
Manual		
IIIM	Skilled manual	Supervisors of manual workers, plumbers, electricians, bus drivers
IV	Partly skilled	Warehousemen, security guards, machine tool operators, care assistants
V	Unskilled	Labourers, cleaners, messengers

Source: National statistics website: www.statistics. gov.uk
Crown copyright material is reproduced with the permission of the controller of HMSO
Reproduced under the terms of the Click-Use Licence

deal of difference between people's life expectancy depending on the class to which they belong. In fact, this difference for men has increased over the years. Between 1972 and 1976 a man from class I could expect to live five and half years longer than a man from class V. By 1997 to 1999, however, a class I man could expect to live nearly seven

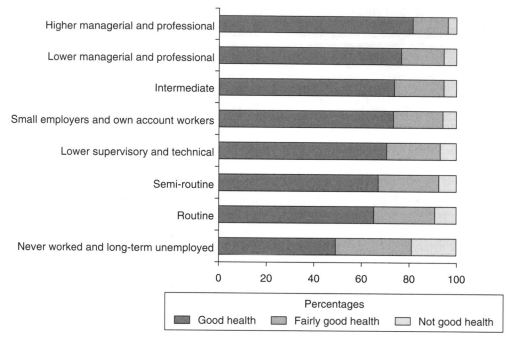

FIGURE 6.2   *Self-reported health by NS-SEC (ONS 2001)*
Source: National Statistics website: www.statistics.gov.uk
Crown copyright material is reproduced with the permission of the Controller of HMSO
Reproduced under the terms of the Click-Use Licence

and a half years longer than a man from class V. In the same period the same difference for women increased from 5.3 years to 5.7 years (ONS 2004: 79).

There are many other ways in which the health, morbidity and mortality of those in the most disadvantaged groups in **society** is worse than those in the most advantaged groups. Another example of this can be found in self-reported health; this is where you ask people to assess how they themselves would rate their health. Again, we find a sharp difference between the classes (see Figure 6.2) , with nearly four times the number of men and women who are long-term unemployed or have never worked rating their health as poor in comparison to men and women in the managerial and professional classification.

Question

How would you assess your health: (a) good (b) fairly good, or (c) not good? How does your assessment of health relate to the statistics mentioned above?

FIGURE 6.3   *All cause death rate: by social class and sex, death rate per 100,000. Men on left side, women on right side (ONS 2004)*
Crown copyright material is reproduced with the permission of the Controller of HMSO
Reproduced under the terms of the Click-Use Licence

One of the clearest ways in which class and health inequalities can be seen is in death rates (see Figure 6.3). Over the last few years the death rate for all classes has dropped but there still remains a distinct class gradient. The gradient tends to be clearer for men but a little more irregular for women. **Gender** differences in health will be explored in more depth in Chapter 8.

Links

Chapter 8 discusses gender and health in more detail.

This pattern of what is known as the 'class and health gradient' is also visible when we look at specific conditions. In just about every case there is greater mortality as we move across the class scale. Figure 6.4 indicates this trend using selected causes of death as examples.

It is just not in physical health that people from classes IV and V exhibit a greater burden of ill health. We can also see it with mental health (see Figure 6.5). There is higher prevalence of many forms of mental ill health among people from classes III Nm, IV and V. Chapter 9 will deal with mental health in much more depth.

Links

Chapter 9 discusses mental health in more detail.

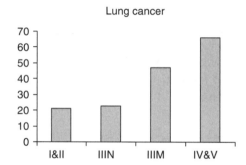

FIGURE 6.4   *Trends in mortality from selected causes of death by social class 1997–99, males aged 35–64, directly age-standardised death rates (DSR) per 100,000 year (ONS 2003)*
Source: National Statistics website: www.statistics.gov.uk
Crown copyright material is reproduced with the permission of the Controller of HMSO
Reproduced under the terms of the Click-Use Licence

Recent work by Shaw et al. (1999) and Dorling et al. (2000) has drawn our attention to how there appears to be some form of relationship between health and place. Bad health is usually found in areas of poverty and deprivation, though there may well be other factors such as environment (how clean the streets are, levels of crime and vandalism, and so on) or access to facilities, for example, which could also contribute to the poor health of certain areas. What Tables 6.3 and 6.4 show is that many of the worst health areas have really high standardised

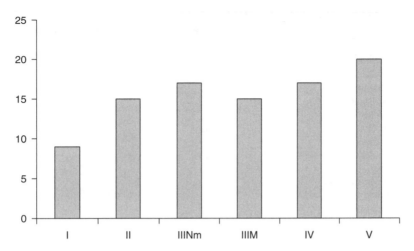

FIGURE 6.5   *Prevalence of neurotic disorders: by social class, 2000. Great Britain, percentages (ONS 2004: 78)*
Source: National Statistics website: www.statistics.gov.uk
Crown copyright material is reproduced with the permission of the Controller of HMSO
Reproduced under the terms of the Click-Use Licence

TABLE 6.3   *Worst health by area in the UK*

Location	SMR	avoidable deaths %
Glasgow Shettleston	234	71
Glasgow Springburn	217	69
Glasgow Maryhill	196	65
Glasgow Pollock	187	64
Glasgow Anniesland	181	63
Glasgow Ballieston	180	62
Manchester Central	174	61
Glasgow Govan	172	61
Liverpool Riverside	172	61
Manchester Blackley	169	60
Greenock and Inverclyde	164	59
Salford	163	59
Tyne Bridge	158	57
Glasgow Kelvin	158	57
Southwark North and Bermondsey	156	56
All	178	62

Source: Shaw et al. 1999
Reproduced by kind permission of The Polity Press

TABLE 6.4   *Best health by area in the UK*

Location	SMR	avoidable deaths %
Wokingham	65	–
Woodspring	65	–
Romsey	65	–
Sheffield Hallam	66	–
South Cambridgeshire	66	–
Chesham and Amersham	67	–
South Norfolk	69	–
West Chelmsford	69	–
South Suffolk	69	–
Witney	69	–
Esher and Walton	69	–
Northavon	70	–
Buckingham	71	–
Total	68	–

Source: Shaw et al. 1999
Reproduced by kind permission of The Polity Press

mortality ratios (SMR), often twice the average. They also have high levels of deaths that would have been avoided had the people not been living in poverty, plus very high levels of child poverty.

It is always worthwhile to reflect on what lies behind these rather cold and stark statistics. What we see here is that there are people living in different parts of the same country, but leading quite different lives in terms of length and quality of life. The numbers of unnecessary deaths can be placed at 10,887 (Smith et al. 2000). Another study into health inequalities and excess mortality (Mitchell et al. 2000) also pointed to the substantial number of lives that could be saved each year if certain changes in **social policy** were made. The potential numbers of lives that could be saved and the policy changes that could bring that about are summarised in Figure 6.6.

No of lives saved per year	Policy change
7,597 among people under 65	If wealth inequalities were reduced to their 1983 level
2,504 among people under 65	If there was full employment
1,407 among those under 15	If child poverty was eradicated
11,508* in total	If all three measures were implemented
*after rounding.	

FIGURE 6.6   *Lives saved by various changes in social policy (Mitchell et al. 2000)*
Reproduced by kind permission of The Polity Press

Question

Shaw et al. (1999) draw our attention to the effect of place. Look at the photographs above of an area that could be associated with deprivation. What do you think it would be like living in such an area? In what ways could your health be affected? In addition to material (quality of housing, for example), what about stress?

The above information may give the impression that there is a 'north–south' divide, with the south being affluent and healthy while the north is poor and unhealthy. One must take care here, as the picture is a little more complex. Poverty and deprivation may be disguised and camouflaged in what, at first glance, appear to be relatively affluent areas. A closer **analysis** of the data and research reveals that there exist pockets of poverty in the south-east where conditions are similar to those found in places such as Glasgow Shettleston. This is illustrated in a report by

Dorling et al. (2000) poverty and health inequality in London. Following Charles Booth's classic study of poverty in London in 1896 (Booth 1902), they found that not much had changed in the last hundred years. Booth's study involved a painstaking house-by-house, street-by-street analysis of poverty and wealth in London. He then produced a colour-coded map indicating the poorest areas in black and the most affluent areas in light yellow. Dorling et al. found that Booth's map still held up as a very powerful indicator of where to find both poverty and ill health. This indicates that even in a relatively prosperous area such as the south-east of England there exist dense pockets of poverty, and that a hundred years of apparent social progress and social policy have produced little change in parts of the UK.

If those 11,508 people had died in a tragic accident in the London Tube or as a result of a mistake made in a hospital procedure, the outcry and national shock would have been overwhelming. However, these people died individually and unnoticed, hidden away in the forgotten housing estates and housing schemes of Britain's main urban areas; the invisible, marginalised and excluded victims of the widening gulf in wealth and health.

Question

Why do you think governments do not make the changes in social policy suggested by Mitchell et al. (2000) that could save the lives of 11,508 people?

6.3 Social inequalities

One feature of contemporary British society is that there are clear and enduring inequalities whether in health (as seen earlier), income or wealth. This section will explore those inequalities further and outline that Britain today is still a very divided and unequal place to live. In particular, we shall look at differences in wealth and income and the associated problems of poverty, before looking at some of the research that sheds light on what it is to live on a limited budget with regard to the ability to afford a decent nutritious diet.

Income and wealth inequality

A clear and persistent trend over the last thirty years or so has been the location of vast amounts of wealth (the money found in shares, savings, artwork, jewellery,

TABLE 6.5   *Distribution of wealth*

	1976	**1986**	**1991**	**1996**	**2001**
Most wealthy 1%	21	18	17	20	23
Most wealthy 2%	71	73	71	74	75
Most wealthy 3%	92	90	92	93	95

Source: National Statistics website: www.statistics.gov.uk
Crown copyright material is reproduced with the permission of the Controller of HMSO
Reproduced under the terms of the Click-Use Licence

land) in the hands of a small percentage of people (see Table 6.5). In fact the wealthiest 1 per cent owns as much wealth as the poorest 50 per cent – a very sizeable inequality!

Inequality is also apparent in income. The highest paid in British society earn ten times as much as the lowest paid in terms of average gross weekly pay, as Table 6.6 indicates.

Poverty remains a pressing issue in today's society in the UK with just under 13 million people living below the poverty line. There are two forms of poverty: **absolute poverty** – the complete absence of clothing, food and shelter, typically seen in developing countries; and **relative poverty** – where people have a standard of living that is lower than an acceptable standard of living in a given society. Relative poverty is the main type that is found in Europe. The European Community offers the following definition of relative poverty:

> Persons, families and groups of persons whose resources (material, cultural and social) are so limited as to exclude them from the minimum acceptable way of life in the Member State to which they belong. (SPIU 1997: 1)

There is a considerable debate as to how and why poverty is defined in certain ways and this has consequences for government policy and action. The Conservative government during the 1980's made the point that there was no poverty in the UK – simply some people with less than others, a feature of any advanced industrial country. This contrasts with Tony Blair's Labour government which sought during the late 1990s and early in the new century to reduce levels of poverty and inequality. There are indications that they have achieved some, albeit limited, success in this regard.

The debates that rage around defining and subsequently measuring poverty are interesting and challenging. It is not, however, within the scope of this section to pursue them in any great depth though a brief consideration will be given below.

So how is poverty measured? There are two main indicators that are used:

- Households below average income (HBAI)
- Income support/job-seekers' allowance levels (IS)

Absolute poverty refers to having such restricted access to food, shelter and clothing that it is life-threatening.
Relative poverty refers to having the minimum requirements of a particular society in relation to other people in that society.

TABLE 6.6   *Top ten highest and lowest average gross weekly incomes*

		Average gross weekly pay (£)
Highest Paid		
1	Directors and chief executives of major organisations	2,301.2
2	Medical practitioners	1,186.4
3	Financial managers and chartered secretaries	1,124.2
4	Solicitors and lawyers, judges and coroners	925.8
5	Marketing and sales managers	888.6
6	Information and communication technology managers	872.4
7	Management consultants, actuaries, economists and statisticians	863.1
8	Police officers (inspectors and above)	863.1
9	IT strategy and planning professionals	844.4
10	Financial and accounting technicians	838.1
Lowest Paid		
1	Retail cashiers and check-out operators	207.6
2	Launderers, dry cleaners, pressers	217.6
3	Bar staff	217.9
4	Waiters, waitresses	218.2
5	Kitchen and catering assistants	228.4
6	Hotel porters	229.9
7	Hairdressers, barbers	231.8
8	Animal care occupations (not elsewhere classified)	232.3
9	Sewing machinists	239.8
10	Shelf fillers	241.5

Source: National Statistics website: www.statistics.gov.uk
Crown copyright material is reproduced with the permission of the Controller of HMSO
Reproduced under the terms of the Click-Use Licence

Households below average income

The first measure relies upon using 50 per cent mean and/or 60 percent median of average income for a particular household (Figure 6.7). The figures, published by the Department of Work and Pensions, review income distribution throughout the UK. The figures are of income *before* and *after* housing costs. However, it is mainly *after*-housing-costs figures that are used because, for poorer people, housing costs are inescapable fixed costs and using after-housing-costs figures provides a more accurate reflection of disposable income. The poverty line using this particular measure is shown in Figure 6.8.

Using this measure of poverty we can chart the growth of poverty since 1979, as Figure 6.7 indicates.

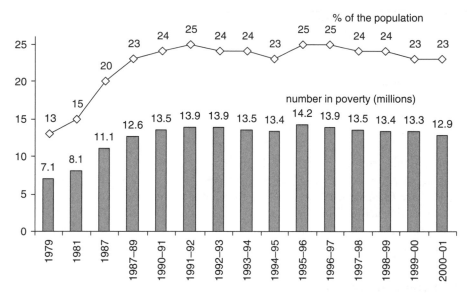

FIGURE 6.7   *The number of households below 60 per cent median income (after housing costs and including self-employed) 1979–2000/01 UK (SPIU 2002)*

The poverty line using income support/income-based jobseeker's allowance, January 2002, £ per week	
Single person aged 18–24	£42.00
Single person aged 25+	£53.05
Couple (both aged 18+)	£83.25
Couple (both 18+ but under 60) with three children aged under 11	£192.10
Lone parent (aged 18+) with one child under 11	£100.50
Single pensioner (aged 60–74)	£92.15
Pensioner Couple (aged 60–74)	£140.55

FIGURE 6.8   *The poverty line using income support/income-based jobseeker's allowance (after housing costs) (SPIU 2002)*

Income support/job-seekers' allowance

The second measure uses benefit levels (see Figure 6.8) as a method of measuring the poverty line. Benefit levels are useful because they indicate an official minimum necessary to subsist, according to the government.

Poverty affects a wide and varied cross-section of the **community**. The follow-ing groups, in particular, are vulnerable to poverty:

- women
- unemployed and low-paid people
- older and retired people
- ethnic minority groups
- disabled people

One particular trend within the UK has been the number of children living in poverty. Around one in three children now lives below the poverty line. In interna-tional terms this puts the UK almost at the top of the table.

As with the defining of poverty there is a great deal of debate as to what causes poverty; arguments rage on one side identifying *structural* reasons while others point to *individual* weakness. These ideas are summarised below.

Structural explanations

Poverty here is seen as the result of government policy and the booms and busts of the global economic system. During the 1980s in the UK the then Conservative government introduced free-market policies that led to a major readjustment of the UK industrial landscape. Many traditional heavy industries, such as coal mining and steel production, went into terminal decline. This resulted in the economic blight of many areas, particularly south Wales and northern England. It should be borne in mind that when a major employer in an area ceases production it is not just that the workers lose their jobs, but that the whole local economy suffers. Shock waves are sent through the local community, resulting in difficulties for the local service sector and small businesses.

Structural explanations of poverty highlight failures of government policy, and fluctuations in global economics as the root cause of poverty.

It was not just changes to industrial policy that led to an increase in poverty. Changes in taxation and policies concerned with the redistribution of wealth also had a major impact on poverty levels, according to this perspective. Again, during the 1980s, we see a dramatic shift taking place in policy direction. The Conservatives pursued polices that saw a move of wealth up the class scale, as opposed to across it.

Individual explanations

Individual explanations of poverty highlight individual weakness, and individuals taking advantage of state benefits. This view of poverty gained prominence during the 1980s and 1990s, championed by commentators such as David Marsland in the UK and Charles Murray in the US. It attributes poverty either to individual weakness or fecklessness, or to people misusing welfare services. Murray developed the notion of an underclass consisting of people who have voluntarily absented themselves from the working world and who instead live on over-generous state benefits. Many adherents of this view called for the introduction of workfare-style policies, whereby eligibility for benefits is dependent on the completion of some form of training or work. Marsland (1996) points to the welfare state as being responsible for creating a 'dependency culture', where there is little incentive to work.

Question

Which of the two different explanations of poverty do you find the more convincing and why?

Experiencing poverty – Diet and nutrition: rational responses to an irrational situation?

Poverty has already been outlined statistically. This is useful and highly informative, but it is also important to understand what day-to-day life is like for someone living in poverty. Let us start by challenging one misconception – that poverty is just a case of tightening one's belt, and budgeting better by, let's say, opting for cheaper foods. Poverty is much more than that as it entails a complete dislocation and reorganising of one's life, with many of the social norms and accepted patterns of cultural life being turned on their head. People are driven to actions which, on the surface, appear to be bad economy or a misuse of limited funds, such as spending money on low-quality, high-fat foods or not buying cheaper bulk goods. However, on closer examination, we find that for many people these are rational responses to an irrational situation. It is illuminating to look at recent research into food-purchasing patterns among those living in poverty.

On one level, statistics indicate that people living in poverty make bad choices when it comes to nutrition, for their diets are often high in processed sugars or fats – ingredients that contribute to heart problems, obesity and the risk of cancer. This raises the possibility that people living in poverty are incapable of making the correct choices because they lack knowledge or information, and therefore many health promotion campaigns aim at encouraging people to eat more vegetables and cut back on fats. However, the situation is perhaps a little more complex.

Dobson et al. (1994) researched forty-eight households, half of which were lone mother families, to investigate food purchasing and attitudes towards eating. What they found was a pattern of life in which food and eating lost most of their pleasurable social and cultural aspects – such as being enjoyable or something shared with friends and families – to be replaced with a strict discipline and constant economic restrictions. When shopping, any notion of experimenting with new or interesting products was put aside and choice limited to cheap brands and to foods that mothers knew would be eaten by their children. This last point is significant as it indicates why some people eat what in other circumstances would be regarded as 'bad' foods. Here mothers bought foods such as crisps or chocolates because they did not want to risk wasting money on foodstuffs their children might not eat. Here we see an example of a rational choice in irrational circumstances. It must also be noted that many of the families did have an awareness of healthy eating but were sceptical about the messages they received or about the costs involved in putting healthy eating into practice.

Other research on food purchasing indicates further difficulties facing those in poverty. The National Children's Homes (1991) survey on nutrition and poverty found that one tactic to minimise household spending is to skip meals altogether. They found that one child in ten and one adult in five skipped meals because of cost. However, it is not only people failing to choose the 'right' foods or opting not to eat for financial reasons, but also the availability of affordable food that is problematic. The National Food Alliance (BBC News 1998) points to the existence of what is termed 'food deserts', inner-city areas where cheap nutritious foods are not available because of the absence of large supermarkets. People in deprived areas have to rely upon corner shops or smaller retail outlets that do not have the same economy of scale as the larger chains, and as a consequence are more expensive. Again we see costs as a contributory factor in limiting choice. Other research has indicated that for poorer people a greater percentage of their budgets is taken up with food purchasing than is the case with those who are better off (Blackburn 1991). What we see here is that financial pressure is increased by having to spend the bulk of available income on attempting to keep body and soul together and maintain an adequate diet.

Overall, poverty affects nutrition in the following ways:

- Choice is affected by limited funds.
- Food loses all social and cultural significance.
- Shopping for food is not a pleasurable experience and reinforces feelings of social exclusion.
- Purchasing 'healthier' options is avoided on the grounds that they may not be eaten, thus wasting already limited funds.
- The existence of food deserts makes it difficult for those living in impoverished areas to access cheap nutritious foods.

- Malnutrition is a problem among certain social classes in contemporary Britain.
- People living in poverty spend a higher percentage of their incomes on food than those who are not.

Question

Think of your own diet – is it what you want it to be? Do you know what a good diet should consist Can you afford to eat nutritious food all the time? In terms of your own budget, do you ever cut back on food to pay for other things?

6.4 Explaining class and health inequalities

So far, we have examined a great deal of material about the disparities that exist in health and income/wealth across different groups. These statistics provide a great deal of information and strongly indicate that class and health inequality exists. Statistics alone, however, are never enough for the **sociological imagination** and we must turn to theories that can explain those statistics. Essentially, we must ask why and how these differences come into existence. What we shall see is that it is more complicated than just that poor people eat unhealthy food options or the rich have access to private health care.

This will be the main purpose of this section: to explore beneath the surface and see what causes so many people to have the length of their lives reduced and experience greater ill-health than others. To do so we will begin by briefly looking at the Black Report, a highly influential piece of work published in 1980, which drew attention to many forms of health inequality in British society.

Attention will then turn to the current debate between two, in many ways rival and competing, theories that seek to explain class and health inequalities: the psycho–social and the neo–material. These theories emphasise different reasons why class and health inequality exists. The *psycho-social* focuses on the negative emotional experiences, the stresses and strains, of living in an unequal society. The *neo-material* favours an explanation that concentrates on the distribution of various resources such as good housing and education.

The Black Report

Published back in 1980, the Black Report (Black et al. 1980) has, in many respects, set the agenda for research into all manner of health inequalities in the UK. Mainly

TABLE 6.7   *Table Summarising Black Report and lessons from subsequent research.*

Suggested reasons for health inequalities	Subsequent research
Artefact explanation	
The existence of health inequalities is due to the way in which the statistics are collected and the way in which we construct class.	If anything, the statistics under-report the extent of class and health inequalities.
Social selection explanation	
It is poor health that assigns people to lower-class groups rather than any of the effects of belonging to a lower class group. Thus it is the other way around, health affects our class, rather than class affecting our health.	There may be some evidence of social selection at younger ages but the overall effect over a lifetime is very minor.
Behavioural/cultural explanations	
Ill health is due to people's choices and decisions; working-class people tend to make the wrong choices to smoke, drink too much and eat the wrong foods.	Even among people who follow 'healthy lifestyles' we find similar patterns of ill-health. Lifestyle choices may only account for a quarter of social-class inequalities.
Structural/material explanations	
Poor conditions, such as bad housing and low incomes, make it virtually impossible for working-class people to lead a healthy lifestyle.	This perspective will be explored in greater depth in the rest of this chapter.

Source: Kirby et al. 1997

drawn from epidemiological research the report identified that there were clear and distinct differences in the health of men and women, ethnic minority groups and between classes. In terms of class, The Black Report put forward four different possible explanations of why class has such a strong bearing on health: artefact, social selection, cultural and material. Over the years these explanations of why class and health inequalities exist have been challenged, modified or developed. However, given the importance of the Black Report at the time it is useful to have an awareness of both the reasons it suggested for health inequalities and what the subsequent research has found. All of this is summarised in Table 6.7.

Psycho-social or neo-material explanations

We will now look at the psycho–social and neo–material explanations that attempt to explain the existence of class and health inequalities. A convenient metaphor for explaining the differences between the two approaches is provided by Lynch et al. (2000). Society is like a passenger plane. There are a few roomy comfortable business class seats at the front while the rest of the plane consists of less spacious economy class seats. From the **psycho–social perspective** the poor health of the economy class passengers is due to them feeling stressed at seeing the comfort of the business class passengers. From the neo-material perspective the health inequality is due to the cramped conditions of their seating.

The psycho-social perspective

Earlier in this chapter, we saw how vast the gap is when it comes to the health of various social classes within the UK. In many ways, this is not only shocking but also surprising, considering how advanced and developed the UK is in comparison with other countries. As already noted, around 10,500 people, one could argue, die as a result of health and poverty inequalities. Intuitively one would think that when a country's economy improved then there would be a resultant increase in life expectancy *and* general health. This assumption was challenged by Wilkinson's (1996) work in the 1980s and 1990s which demonstrated that in affluent societies it is *relative*, not *average*, income that affects health. What Wilkinson essentially argues is that the greater the inequality in a given society, the less social cohesion it has and, therefore, the more insecurity and isolation experienced by the most disadvantaged groups in that society. This insecurity and isolation result in greater levels of chronic stress. In turn, this chronic stress moves down biological pathways (particularly the nervous system) in the human body causing all sorts of harm.

Using one of Wilkinson's (1996: 86) examples we can see his wider point. If we compare the UK to other countries we come across some interesting observations. A comparison of the class and mortality rates between England and Wales and Sweden provides a notable example, and is useful since Sweden and the UK are both affluent Western European nations. England and Wales exhibit sharp differences between the social classes, while for Sweden those differences are marginal. Wilkinson (1996) suggests this is because of greater income equality in Sweden. He goes on to comment that if England and Wales had similar income distribution patterns to that of Sweden there would be a dramatic improvement in the health of those in the lower social classes. It is also noticeable that the lowest social group in Sweden has a better mortality rate than that of the highest in England and Wales – so greater income equality would benefit not just the most deprived groups, but everybody.

This raises a related question about wider inequalities in society. Marmot (1986), when investigating the health of civil servants who worked in Whitehall, makes some interesting points. Marmot found that lower-grade civil servants suffered worse health than higher-grade civil servants. This again indicates that social divisions or the existence of hierarchies can have an adverse effect on health. More recent work by Marmot's colleagues Bosma et al. (1997) and Martikainen et al. (1999) supports the idea that the stress created by inequality also negatively affects health in the workplace.

Psycho-social perspectives refer to explanations of class and health inequality that emphasise the negative emotional experiences of living in an unequal society, particularly feelings of stress, shame and powerlessness. **Neo-material perspectives** refer to explanations of class and health inequality that emphasise unequal distribution of resources such as housing, income and access to education.

So we have seen how inequality and a society with sizeable gaps between the rich and the poor can lead to worse health for everyone, but particularly for those at the lower end of the social scale. This raises the question: what are the characteristics of a healthy society? Wilkinson (1996) points to societies that exhibit high social cohesion. These societies are characterised by mutual aid, narrow differences in income and a shared sense of purpose or belief. There exist several examples of societies that exhibit these characteristics, but the two that will be discussed in greater detail are Britain during the war years, and Roseto, Pennsylvania, USA.

Both the First and Second World Wars are remembered with a multitude of complementary and contradictory images. One thinks of both the heroism and tragedy of the First World War, and the triumph over Fascism but also the Holocaust of the Second. Many of the images relate to privation, to people losing their homes in bombing raids or difficulties caused by shortages of various kinds. Nevertheless, one interesting fact emerges from the war years – the health of nation improved! The greatest increases in life expectancy occurred during the war years. So how did this happen? One might expect it to be the introduction of rationing, whereby everyone could access a decent diet. Before rationing, the diet of many working-class people was very restricted and deficient in vegetables and meat. However, there was no rationing during the First World War. Wilkinson (1996) suggests that the narrowing of income differences, the reduction in poverty, and a sense of social solidarity were more likely to have influenced this increase in life expectancy. Here we see an example of how people who live in a more egalitarian society, with a common sense of identity and of purpose, are healthier.

Social cohesion implies feeling part of a society or social group; often this is expressed through helping others, and placing emphasis on the group as opposed to the individual. It is this feeling part of something that helps people to be healthier.

Question

Wilkinson argues that social cohesion makes for better health, but just how socially cohesive is society today? Reflect on your circumstances and think about how often neighbours help each other or people gather together for social events.

Roseto is a classic example of how social cohesion affects the health of people in a particular community. Research by Bruhn and Wolf (1979) has identified a very interesting relationship between the changing culture of the town and the health of its citizens. The town, situated in eastern Pennsylvania, was founded by Italian migrants in the 1880s. It was noticeably healthier than its neighbouring towns, with markedly lower death rates even in the mid-1930s, especially from heart disease, which was 40 per cent lower. This was not due to factors such as diet, smoking or exercise. The diet of the people who lived there was very high in saturated fats, particularly lard. The reasons for this good health are, rather, attributable to social factors.

Neighbouring towns noted that Roseto, from its foundation, had a strong sense of social cohesion underpinned by a very egalitarian approach to life. There was a uniformity about the people, who eschewed any notions of competing with their neighbours; indeed there was a strong emphasis on the family and on helping neighbours. Bruhn and Wolf concluded that this acted as a strong protective factor against heart disease. However, as time passed, those original founding values were replaced by the more competitive individualistic culture of mainstream America. As a consequence, the protective effects of social cohesion and egalitarianism were lost and the health advantage disappeared.

Work in the UK has revealed a similar picture where people are supported and are part of a cohesive community. Oakley and Rajan (1991) investigated social class and social support in relation to young pregnant women. Their findings were interesting for two reasons. First, they argued that the traditional idea that community and social cohesion were working-class phenomena was misplaced. It was mainly middle-class women who had a network of supportive social contacts. This led to their second finding, that the women who had supportive relationships with others gave birth to heavier, healthier babies. Again, we see the usefulness of some form of social contact as a way of predicting better health.

Wilkinson also provides us with a pathway of how social inequality and chronic stress lead to biological disturbance and consequently bad health. As part of our biological make-up, we humans, like other animals, possess what is commonly known as a 'flight-or-fight' mechanism, which protects us against things that could potentially harms us. This is something we acquired during our evolution and throughout human history it was very necessary for our preservation. Essentially, when we are confronted by, let's say, a lion on the African savannah our body reacts by releasing certain stress chemicals. These stress chemicals, particularly cortisol, make the body act in certain ways so that we are at our physical best to either run away (the flight option) or attack the lion (the fight option). In doing so, these chemicals stop other parts of our physiological system (the immune system and tissue repair, for example) from working. This is intended to be a temporary measure with everything focused on improving the body's performance to deal with whatever is stressing us. In modern industrial societies, however, the type of stress we encounter is different from the type of stress caused by unexpectedly meeting a lion. The stress we encounter, for example a busy unending workload, often tends to be prolonged. Our stress reactions still kick in, though. Crucially, this time instead of being temporary, the shut-down of the immune system and tissue repair lasts a long time. Thus, our ability to deal with infection is greatly weakened and the general biological maintenance of our bodies does not take place. Also, the extended presence of cortisol can have very damaging effects on the body.

The neo-material perspective

Wilkinson's theories of social cohesion have animated a great deal of at times quite heated debate. Some, such as Judge et al. (1997), have taken him to task for the way he has marshalled empirical evidence to support his overall argument. One of the most stringent criticisms has come from Lynch and colleagues who have proposed a neo-material explanation in contrast to Wilkinson's psycho-social perspective. Though having some sympathy with the general idea that unequal societies produce stress they argue that Wilkinson ignores material factors such as educational disadvantage, poor housing, availability of healthy food and access to decent social welfare.

More generally the neo-materialists (Lynch et al. 2000: 1202) have four further objections to Wilkinson's psycho-social perspective:

- The structural causes of inequality are insufficiently recognised in the psycho-social explanation. The actual reasons why inequalities exist in the first place is not addressed or explained, suggesting that they are of lesser importance.
- One must be careful in seeing tight-knit communities as inherently a good thing: sometimes social bonds can be a source of stress or discrimination against others or minority groups.
- Focusing on social cohesion at a community level takes no account of how larger social institutions and structures, such as the government or the economy, affect and influence the conditions that either help or hinder social cohesion.
- Again, by just focussing on social cohesion, the wider political context is ignored. Though, not intended by those who support the psycho-social perspective, this could lead to victim blaming, allowing governments to claim that the reason for poor health is that the community is at fault for having poor social cohesion.

Coburn (2000, 2004) has added to the debate by arguing that we must also be aware of and take into account deeper forces at play in the economy and in society. In particular, he draws our attention to the effect of neo-liberalism both on widening class differences and consequently on the health of working-class people. He claims that the political, social and economic policies followed by many of the world's major countries (but mainly the US and the UK) lead to an increase in social inequalities in income and wealth, in addition to an increasing individualism that works against social cohesion.

Question

We have now looked at the two current competing perspectives. Which one do you find the more convincing and why?

Conclusion

The research presented here clearly indicates that there are consistent and persistent differences in class and health in contemporary society. Such differences are part of the array of inequalities to do with wealth, income and other resources. Perhaps it is in health that the social division of class is most evidently visible, with the bodies of people affected and changed by their location in society. The bodies of working-class people are more likely to age quicker, be more susceptible to illness and be much more likely to encounter limiting long-term conditions than those located higher in society. The evidence also strongly points to these health differences being explainable not purely as the result of the actions and choices made by individual people but by deep impersonal structural forces (for example poverty, income differences and access to resources) that are beyond their control.

Exactly, how best to explain those differences is still open to debate. Currently, the focus is on whether it is psycho-social or neo-material explanations that offer the best theoretical articulation of class and health inequalities. Each places an emphasis on different causes, whether it is to do with the experiences of living in an unequal society or to the iniquitous distribution of the resources that are necessary for good health. It may be that the two explanations could be 'combined' (as indicated by some commentators, such as Yuill 2005 and Williams 2003) to explain different aspects of health inequalities – though this would require considerable refining and clarifying of important points. This could allow us to see what causes inequalities in the first place (best explained by the neo-material explanation) and how those inequalities are experienced in everyday life (best explained by the psycho-social explanation). This is possibly where the sociology of class and health inequalities could go next, but one point appears certain: as long as a class society exists, so too will health inequalities.

SUMMARY POINTS

- Class is a complex and dynamic power relationship between people.
- Class differences can be measured statistically using two different methods: the Registrar-General's Social Class scheme and the National Statistics Socio-economic Classification.
- A man from social class I lives on average 7.4 years longer than a man from social class V. For women the difference is 5.7 years.
- For self-reported health those from the most advantaged groups indicate higher levels of good health and lower levels of poor health than the least advantaged groups.
- Across just about every cause of early mortality both class V men and women will exhibit higher levels of early death than men and women from class I.
- Mental health problems also affect a higher number of people from classes IV and V than from classes I and II.
- There exists considerable class inequality in the UK today.
- Poverty continues to be a social problem: though the situation is better than it was, poverty in the UK is still worse than in other European countries.
- There have been several attempts over the years to explain class and health inequalities.
- The classic Black Report looked at material, behavioural, cultural and artefact explanations.
- Current explanations centre on the psycho-social versus the neo-material explanations.
- The psycho-social approach draws our attention to the stress of living in an unequal society.
- The neo-material approach draws our attention to the uneven distribution of resources.

Case study

The following extract is from David Widgery's (1991) book reflecting on his experiences as a GP working in the East End of London. Throughout, Widgery conveys the hopelessness and tragedy of hundreds of lives wasted and worn out by the grinding poverty that he sees on a daily basis, whether in his surgery or on home visits. His experiences are common to most GPs working in what are termed 'deprived areas'.

The following extract is from a chapter of impressionistic notes made after a typical day visiting various patients, hence their rather hurried nature.

Back pain at midnight. Single seventeen-year-old in squat. Beside bed a signed photo. Not her boyfriend, a male stripper she had met the previous night. Virtually no possessions but emerged each morning in immaculate eye make-up and leather miniskirt. She'd fallen over in her mayonnaise factory. Says she works in puddles of pickle juice and oil. Later her child goes into care because of heroin. Looked after a woman dealer's dogs and got paid in heroin. 'But I shopped her, the cow.' She comes back occasionally, after dihydrocodeine.

Patients with high anxiety, low expectations. Exhibitionists: wrist slashers, plate throwers, overdose artists. Manic depressive with bits of paper. … Odd, unmatching clothes (sign of Sally Army). Rants off, slamming door. Demented old lady with flat but no carpets. Cupboards but no food, aroma of corned beef, piss and scorched nylon. Full of fury: at the relatives, who had 'deserted' her, the social worker and me …

New patients with impossible demands, old faces with familiar problems. Batty girl: 'The paper in my head tells me to love you.' Entering old, gloomily lit areas of social disorganisation, homes where logic seems to have gone missing. Bare room: bar fire, meter, TV; many high-heeled shoes, about forty pairs! 'Keeping the vodka to one bottle a day, Doc,' she says and falls over.

1   What sort of society do David Widgery's notes describe?
2   How would supporters of (a) the social cohesion or (b) the neo-material approach analyse the lives of the people in the above extract?
3   How would you feel, as a health professional, working in an area like the East End of London as Widgery describes?
4   What could be done to relieve class and health inequalities?

Taking your studies further

This chapter will have helped you understand many of the key terms, concepts, theories and debates relating to class and health. Listed below are journal articles and books that will provide deeper and more detailed discussions of the points raised in this chapter. You will also find what is available on the companion website. This offers downloads of relevant material, plus links to useful websites in addition to podcasts and other features.

Recommended reading

Books

Scambler, G. (2002) *Health and Social Change: A Critical Theory*. Buckingham: Open University Press.

Shaw, M., Dorling, D., Gordon, D. and Davey-Smith, G. (1999) *The Widening Gap: Health Inequalities and Policy in Britain*. Bristol: The Policy Press.

Wilkinson, R.G. (2005) *The Impact of Inequality: How to Make Sick Societies Healthier*. London: Routledge.

Journal articles

Elstad, J.I. (1998) 'The psycho-social perspective on social inequalities in health', *Sociology of Health and Illness*, 20 (5): 598–618.

Marmot, M., Ryff, C.D., Bumpass, L.L., Shipley, M. and Marks, N.F. (1997) 'Social inequalities in health: next questions and converging evidence', *Social Science and Medicine*, 44 (6): 901–10.

Muntaner, C. and Lynch, J. (1999) 'Income inequality, social cohesion, and class relations: a critique of Wilkinson's neo-Durkheimian research program', *International Journal of Health Services*, 29 (1): 59–81.

A useful selection of articles on class and health inequalities can be found in *Social Science and Medicine*, 51 (7) (2000).

Websites

Scottish Poverty Information Unit (SPIU) http://www.povertyinformation.org/

On the companion website

Williams, S.J. (2003) *Medicine and the Body*. London: Sage. Chapter 2 on '"Structuring" bodies: emotions, inequalities and health'.

7

Ethnicity, 'race' and health

MAIN POINTS

- Many countries in Europe and North America are becoming increasingly multicultural.
- Research indicates that ethnic minority groups display an ill-health burden. This is despite many ethnic groups having a younger age profile than the majority White population.
- The reasons for this burden of ill-health mainly relate to socio-economic factors, the effects of racism and negative experiences of medical and health services rather than a genetic or cultural explanation.
- People from ethnic minority groups are more likely to have lower paid and more insecure jobs, worse housing and greater chances of being in poverty than the White majority population.
- Racism is a common and defining experience for many ethnic minority people. The stress of this has a negative impact on health.
- Medical and health services can discriminate against ethnic minority people by providing either insensitive or inappropriate treatment.

KEY CONCEPTS

'Race', racism, ethnicity, prejudice, discrimination, sterotypes, institutional racism.

Introduction

Events such as 9/11, the ensuing 'War on Terror', migration from the new member states of the European Union, and the success of far-right political parties also across Europe has led to a strong focus on issues of **ethnicity** and identity in the opening decade of this century. Much of this is the consequence of increasing globalisation, which has seen both the movements not just of consumer goods but also of people. This, on one hand, brings about a richer more diverse culture, with different traditions and ways of life fusing into new exciting forms, notably in the fields of fashion, music and food. To that end Beck (2002: 28) has commented that, 'world society has taken possession of our kitchens and is boiling and sizzling in our pans'. These are very positive contemporary examples of ethnicity and culture. On the other hand, there have been less positive developments. In the wake of the 9/11 and 7/7 attacks there has been an increase in 'Islamophobia', and the rise of far-right parties across Europe.

This chapter will focus on how ethnicity, in our global and fast-changing world, influences health and the variety of complexities that go with looking at such a sensitive area. There has been much research on ethnicity and health over the years. What much of the research indicates is that there is a burden of ill-health among ethnic minority groups in the UK. Many people from ethnic minority groups report poor health and long-term limiting illness (see Figure 7.1). This is even more notable as ethnic minority groups tend to have a younger age profile than the White majority population. Summarising trends from the Fourth National Survey of Ethnic Minorities of ethnic minority groups in England and Wales Nazroo (1997: 32) noted the following:

- One in three reported less than good health, or long-standing illness or that they were registered disabled.
- Almost one in six reported that their health limited their performance of moderate activities, or climbing one flight of stairs, or walking half a mile or carrying groceries.
- One in 25 reported a diagnosis of heart disease, while among those aged 40 or older, one in ten reported a diagnosis of heart disease and almost one in six reported a diagnosis or symptoms suggestive of heart disease.
- One in ten reported a diagnosis of hypertension.
- One in 20 reported a diagnosis of diabetes.
- Almost one in five reported symptoms suggestive of respiratory disease. (Nazroo, 1997: 32)

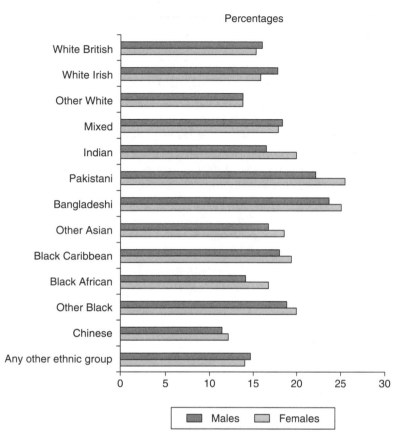

FIGURE 7.1   *Age-standardised limiting long-term illness: by ethnic group and sex, April 2001, England and Wales (National Statistics website: www.statistics.gov.uk)*
Source: National Statistics website: www.statistics.gov.uk
Crown copyright material is reproduced with the permission of the Controller of HMSO
Reproduced under the terms of the Click-Use Licence

Researchers in the past often favoured explanations that drew attention to either genetic or cultural reasons for ill-health. The implication was that there was something wrong with the biology of ethnic groups, which predisposed them to certain types of ill-health or that the culture of the ethnic group was to blame. An indicative example of this older approach can be noted in research on 'South Asians' and coronary heart disease (CHD) (Nazroo 1998). Work by Gupta et al. (1995) inferred that it was something to do with either the genetic make-up of 'South Asians' that predisposed them to CHD, or something in cultural practices such as cooking with ghee, not exercising or not making the best use of medical services. Part of the reason why this 'victim blaming' came about was the research method used. Drawing on certain statistical and quantitative approaches, ethnicity here was treated in a stereotypical manner casting all 'South Asians' as genetically and culturally identical. Such approaches also ignored the socio-economic context in which 'South Asian' people found themselves, for example **class** and the effects of poorly paid jobs. Fenton and Charsley (2000) point out that the complexities, subtleties and sensitivities of understanding ethnicity are often ignored, or not fully appreciated, by the older positivist approaches. In the past few years, however, the work of other researchers, such as Ahmad (2000), Nazroo (2006) and Smaje (1996), have put forward a more challenging and sophisticated explanation of the complex way in which ethnicity, **society** and health interact. As Higginbottom (2006: 585) usefully summarises, variations in ethnicity and health and ill-health, 'arise from the coalescence of complex factors such as migration, cultural adaptation, **racism**, reception by the host **community**, socio-economic influences and prevailing societal ideologies'. In this chapter we will look closely at how the health of ethnic minority groups is adversely affected by social context (socio-economic position, **gender** and racism) and not by faults in genes or culture.

> **Links**
>
> See Chapter 5 for more information on research methods.

7.1 Demographics

Western European countries are becoming increasingly multicultural and, in many ways, Britain is one of the most multicultural with a substantial and diverse ethnic population. Though a great deal of ethnic minority migration into Britain happened in the 1950s, it is worth pointing out that there has been some form of ethnic population in Britain for centuries. We can find evidence of a Black and Asian presence dating back to Roman times in Britain. Black North Africans who had been serving in Rome's Legions in the third century AD lived and settled near Wallsend after finishing their time in the Roman army. Britain between AD 193 and 211 was ruled by the Black Roman Emperor, Septimus Severius, who died in York and was cremated there at a time when York was the capital of Roman Britain. There are other examples throughout history and one has to remember that in the era of slavery

IMAGE 7.1   *The grave of Scipio Africanus (Photograph courtesy of William Avery)*
This image was sourced from:
http://commons.wikimedia.org/wiki/Image:Scipio_Africanus_grave.jpg
From there it can be further used and distributed

there was a Black population in Britain. For example, in St Mary's churchyard in Henbury near Bristol lies the grave of Scipio Africanus who died near there in 1720 aged 18 (see image 7.1).

Question

Does it surprise you to learn that there has been a long history of Black people in Britain? What does such information make you think about what it means to be British?

In Britain the 2001 national census revealed that 7.9 per cent of the population come from a non–White ethnic group (ONS 2005). For the first time ever, a Mixed

TABLE 7.1   *Population: by ethnic group, April 2001 (ONS 2005b: 1)*

	Numbers	Total population (percentages)	Non-White population (percentages)
White	54,153,898	92.1	–
Mixed	677,117	1.2	14.6
Indian	1,053,411	1.8	22.7
Pakistani	747,285	1.3	16.1
Bangladeshi	283,063	0.5	6.1
Other Asian	247,664	0.4	5.3
All Asian or Asian British	2,331,423	4.0	50.3
Black Caribbean	565,876	1.0	12.2
Black African	485,277	0.8	10.5
Black other	97,585	0.2	2.1
All Black or Black British	1,148,738	2.0	24.8
Chinese	247,403	0.4	5.3
Other ethnic groups	230,615	0.4	5.0
All minority ethnic population	4,635,296	7.9	100.0
All population	58,789,194	100.0	

Source: National Statistics website: www.statistics.gov.uk
Crown copyright material is reproduced with the permission of the Controller of HMSO
Reproduced under the terms of the Click-Use Licence

option was included in the census to reflect the increasing number of people in the UK who have parents from different ethnic backgrounds. The exact breakdown of population by ethnic group is laid out in Table 7.1 with the make-up of the non-White population shown in Figure 7.2.

7.2 'Race', racism and ethnicity: definitions, debates and issues

Issues of '**race**' and ethnicity are complex and challenging to explore in any field of **sociology**. This is, as we shall see, due to the contentious and, sometimes, political nature of how we define and perceive supposed differences between people. In this section we shall explore the difficulties in how seeing the world as composed of different 'races' is highly problematic and ultimately false. We will also look at how racism develops out of historical and social influences.

Finally, we will question what can appear to be the relatively neutral concept of ethnicity, and point out that it too has several drawbacks.

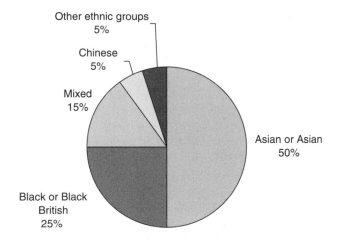

FIGURE 7.2   *The non-White population: by ethnic group, April 2001 (ONS 2005b: 1)*
Source: National Statistics website: www.statistics.gov.uk
Crown copyright material is reproduced with the permission of the Controller of HMSO
Reproduced under the terms of the Click-Use Licence

'Race'

One aspect of modern life is that skin colour is often accepted or regarded as being a major way of seeing differences between people. This follows on from the idea that humanity consists of different 'races', in which there exist discernible and enduring genetic and cultural patterns that clearly separate one group of humans from an other. This can be referred to as an 'essentialist' perspective, where certain traits are seen as naturally given and outside social and historical influence. This implies that things are fixed and that people are born in a certain way that is with them for life. From a sociological perspective, however, this particular view can be challenged and shown to be false. We can also see how such a view is heavily influenced by racist prejudice and stereotyping.

First of all, can classifying humans into separate races be scientifically justified? The concept of 'race' implies that there are different species of people, just as there are different species of animal. The scientific evidence indicates that there exist virtually no major differences between groups of humans. Biologist Steven Rose usefully summarises the genetic science as follows:

The definition of race is essentially a social one, as in reference to Blacks or Jews. While there are differences in gene frequencies (that is, differences in the proportions in which particular genetic variants occur) between population groups, these do not map onto the social criteria used to define race. For instance, Polish Jews resemble genetically their fellow Polish nationals, non-Jews, more closely than they do Jews from Spain. Gene frequencies in Black Americans differ from those in Black South Africans. And that for that matter, gene frequencies differ between people in North and South Wales, yet no one would think of classifying those two populations as two different races. This typological thinking has not disappeared: it characterizes, of course, the poisonous propaganda of racist political groups, and has not entirely vanished from popular scientific writing. (Rose 2005: 37)

What Rose is saying here is that people, regardless of exterior markers such as skin colour, are almost identical. Humans, as a life form, are fairly genetically homogenous and one is likely to find more difference between people who are seen, or see themselves, as, let us say, Asian than between Asian people and people who are seen, or see themselves, as, let us say, White. This is not surprising as in evolutionary time *Homo sapiens* is comparatively recent, emerging out of Africa only c. 200,000 years ago. Simply not enough time to evolve into different groups, species or 'races'!

Rather than seeing differences between humans as being essential or natural we must look to how differences are *socially* constructed over time and in different societies. The whole tradition of thinking in terms of 'race' has a distinct history that is mired in prejudice and oppression. It also emerges out of specific historical and social circumstances. Using skin colour, or 'race', as a delimiter, or way of distinguishing one group of people from another, is historically recent. The first attempt to 'scientifically' classify people did not happen until the mid-1800s. This was the work of De Gobineau and was, at best, based on flimsy pseudo-science and carries no validity today. However, we must look a little further back in time to the rise and expansion of European colonialism and slavery from the mid-1600s to early 1800s. As Blackburn (1998) has discussed, the need for cheap mass labour to work the new plantations in the Americas and the Caribbean led to the enslavement of millions of Black Africans. The sheer brutal and bloody exploitation required some form of justification both on the plantations and in Britain, with many White working-class movements in Britain, such as Chartism, opposed to slavery. So, starting as an oral tradition on the plantations, before becoming part of mainstream European thought, the racist idea that Black people were of a lower order, perhaps even sub-human and therefore not allowed full human rights, spread and developed as part of this process of justifying the slave trade.

Prior to that period, the main ways of seeing differences between people have varied considerably over time. In the ancient world of Rome, Greece and Egypt race and skin colour were not seen as important: instead the world was divided into civilised people and barbarians. Notably, what constituted being civilised was independent of skin colour, with barbarians including White Northern European people and civilised people including Black North Africans. As mentioned before, key historical figures, such as the Roman Emperor Septimus Severius, were Black. Indeed much of the culture of the ancient world to varying degrees was, as Bernal (1991, 2001) has argued, a fusion of European, North African and Asian influences.

Race refers to biological differences between people based on skin colour and other physical features, though the actual differences between them genetically are extremely small. **Ethnicity** refers to the cultural heritage and identity of a group of people. **Racism** refers to the supposed racial superiority of one group over another.

How slaves were stowed in the Brookes of Liverpool. The men's room (C) is to the right, the women's room (G) to the left, and the boys' room (E) in the center. The upper illustration shows the six-foot-wide platform on which slaves were ranged "like books on a shelf"; they had not space above them to sit up. The deck itself (lower illustration) was completely covered with rows of bodies. (From Clarkson's *Abstract of the Evidence*, 1791)

IMAGE 7.2   *Anti-slavery leaflet from 1789*

Image 7.2 is taken from an abolitionist anti-slavery leaflet from 1789. It illustrates the brutal and inhumane way in which enslaved Africans were transported from Africa to the Americas. People were chained to platforms for weeks on end with no access to toilets or fresh air. Millions of Africans died on this transatlantic journey. British ports such as Bristol, Liverpool and Glasgow both directly and indirectly benefited from this trade.

Eamonn is one of the UK's fastest expanding ethnic minority groups. Born in Scotland, he is of Mixed heritage with a White Irish mother and a Black African father. In future years he will have an array of ethnic identities to adopt. He could choose, for example, to call himself Scottish or Black Scottish or maybe Black or Black British. Or perhaps he might prefer Irish or African. In fact, he has a large number of ethnic identities he could choose and then discard throughout his life. Any ethnic identity he may select will be alongside other aspects of his identity too. For example, he'll be someone's son, someone's partner and so on.

Ethnicity

Given the problems associated with 'race', the concept of ethnicity is favoured today. With ethnicity there is no essential basis, no reference to supposed biological or genetic traits, but rather to purely *social* phenomena. Ethnicity refers to a common cultural heritage that is socially learned and constructed. This means that as we grow up we take up and internalise what we see happening about us. So one sees certain ways of dressing and eating, for example, as being normal and adopts them as one's own.

In many respects the concept of ethnicity is a useful advance on, and correction to, the problems of 'race', with its emphasis on the social as opposed to the biological. However, ethnicity too can be problematic. We shall now look at how this is so, considering two main problems in the way that it can sometimes be (mis)used.

Question

To which ethnic group, if any, do you regard yourself as belonging? What are the features (for example, dress, language, food, religion etc.) of your ethnic group? How much of a role, if any, does your ethnicity play in how you see yourself?

Static or fluid?

Ethnicity can be misused in a way that reduces culture to a static list of attributes, with the assumption that everyone who is identified as being in a particular ethnic group shares the same characteristics with regard to, for example, family, life, culture, food, and attitudes to illness and health services. This is seeing ethnicity as being like a shopping list or a 'cookie cutter', where everyone turns out the same. Ethnicity is far more complex than that. One of its complexities is that, like other forms of identity, it is dynamic, evolving and changing over time (Jenkins 2004).

It is useful here to mention that in the wider sociological literature on identity the idea of a fixed static identity is clearly rejected (Giddens 1991; Hall et al. 1993). What is emphasised is that identity is fluid. This means that we can switch between different identities (for example, being British or English, student or therapist, member of a youth subculture or churchgoer) depending on the context we find ourselves in and how we wish to present ourselves. In mainstream culture in the UK we see many examples of both the fluidity and fusion of different ethnic cultures. Programmes like *Goodness Gracious Me* played around with Asian and British stereotypes and introduced many new expressions into the English language, contributing to a way of speaking known as Hinglish.

Atkin et al. (2002) provide a useful example, in relation to disability, of these complexities and of how other forms of identity, in addition to an ethnic identity, can be important in deciding how people perceive themselves in society. Researching how South Asian deaf people negotiate their identity, Ahmad et al. found that the people

TABLE 7.2   *Changes in Scottish identity in relation to British identity 1992–2001*

	1992	**1997**	**1998**	**1999**	**2000**	**2001**
Scottish not British	19	23	32	32	37	36
More Scottish than British	40	38	32	35	31	30
Equal	33	27	28	22	21	24
More British than Scottish	3	4	3	3	3	3
British	3	4	3	4	4	3
None	1	2	2	4	4	4

Source: Bond and Rosie 2002

in their study did not see themselves in a singular way. Rather, the people in the study subscribed to a variety of identities depending on context. These multiple identities ranged from seeing their identity as part of a wider deaf community, to religious identities and to a fusion of British and Asian identities.

Another useful example, this time concerning ethnic identity generally, is how Caribbean migrants thought of their identity in the late 1940s and how it has changed over time. Many early migrants, regardless of which Caribbean island they were originally from, did not see themselves as African-Caribbean (the currently preferred term), but as being British. The following quote is from someone who arrived on the *Empire Windrush* in 1948, as part of the initial phase of migration from the Caribbean into Britain:

'I wouldn't say that we had our own identity. We were always British. In Jamaica I can remember, when it was the Queen's birthday or the King's birthday or the Coronation, everything was done the way Britain wanted us to.' (From Phillips and Phillips 1999: 12)

A unified and distinct African-Caribbean identity developed in Britain in response to the sometime less than welcoming reception that early migrants encountered.

We can see the same fluidity and movement when it comes to ethnic majority identity – an area that is often forgotten about when it comes to matters of ethnicity and health! Bond and Rosie's (2002) work on Scottish identity also demonstrates the lack of a fixed idea of how Scottish people see themselves in relation to an overall British identity (see Table 7.2).

Question

The above discussion talks a lot about fluidity, change and fusion. Identify ways in which both mainstream culture and your own personal life display elements of that fluidity and fusion. You may wish to think about TV programmes, dress, food and so on. Also, why is it important to be aware and knowledgeable about other cultures and ethnicities?

Ethnicity as too general

There is another distinct problem with ethnicity as a concept and how it can be used. The terms used in the UK, such as 'South Asian', are very loose and wide ranging in their coverage. South Asian, for instance, covers a huge geographic range with a population of millions, including India, Sri Lanka, Bangladesh and Pakistan. It also includes a variety of major languages (Punjabi, Gujarati, Pashto, Bengali, Urdu and English) and major religions (Hindu, Islam, Sikh and Christian). Such terms lack any real specificity and can miss out many important and telling differences within an ethnic group. This was suggested by Nazroo (1998) after breaking down the ethnic identity of 'Indian' into religious groups. He found that there were some differences in the reporting of fair or poor health. Indian Hindus, on average, reported similar levels, and Indian Christians slightly better, than the majority White population, while Indian Muslims reported, on average, worse health than all the previously mentioned groups. In the US, Zsembik and Fennell (2005) have drawn attention to the difficulties associated with the concept of a Latino category. Here, again, a variety of people, also from a large and varied land mass, are brought together under one overarching heading. Zsembik and Fennell identify considerable and notable differences in culture, perceptions of health, social class and acculturation for different Latino people. So instead of this one overarching title of Latino, it would be more effective to break it down to identify Mexicans, Puerto Ricans, Dominicans and Cubans as separate groups.

Racism

Even though we have rejected the validity of 'race' as being soundly based in any real science this does not mean that we can reject 'racism' as a force in society just because is based on faulty science (Bradby 1995). Racism is a defining experience for many ethnic groups in the UK, US and elsewhere. As a concept it refers to one group holding itself to be inferior or superior to another group. Earlier we saw that ideas of 'race' and racial superiority developed out of slavery and European colonial expansion. Even though the plantation system, which prompted the emergence of thinking in terms of White superiority over other groups of people, has disappeared racism and all its problems still carry on today. Figure 7.3 indicates that racism is still perceived as a problem in Britain today by a variety of ethnic groups. The current climate of the 'War on Terror' and wider conflicts in the Middle East have also increased tensions concerning Muslims in western countries.

The actual manifestation of racism and the form it takes in society has changed over time, though arguably the result is the same: the systematic disadvantaging of specific minority groups. In the early days of the slave trade racism centred on the supposed sub-human nature of enslaved African people, with claims that they were

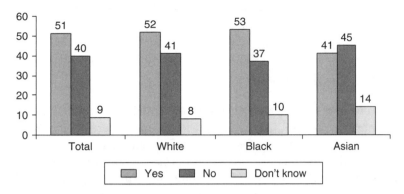

FIGURE 7.3   *ICM poll for the BBC asking 'Do you think Britain is a racist society?'*
Source: BBC (2002)
Reproduced by kind permission of the BBC

a lesser species of humans than white Europeans, and inferior to them in just about any conceivable way. At the high point of the British Empire in the late 1800s racism took on a paternalistic form with notions that colonised peoples required the guidance and help of supposedly more advanced and enlightened Europeans. During the 1980s racism became more disguised and subtle, with the emphasis being on how the survival of indigenous British culture could be overwhelmed by the cultures of migrant ethnic groups. Prime Minister Margaret Thatcher, at the time, went as far as saying that British culture would be 'swamped' by the new groups arriving in the UK. In the wake of the September 11 attack in 2001 on New York and the ensuing 'War on Terror', 'Islamophobia' has been on the rise, with Muslims often portrayed as a potential threat, or having to justify aspects of Islamic culture in a way that other minority ethnic groups are not required to do.

Racism consists of three dimensions. Firstly, there is **prejudice**, which relates to negative attitudes. In a day-to-day context this would mean name-calling on the street and putting forward opinions that denigrate an ethnic group. Next, there is **discrimination**, which relates to actions based on prejudice. This could mean, for example, preventing someone of an ethnic group from getting a job. Research by Noon (1993), for example, found that employers were less likely to employ someone with a typically Asian name than someone with a typically British name. Finally, in recent years in the UK one of the most highlighted and debated forms of racism has been **institutional racism**. The main focus on institutional racism has been in the wake of the MacPherson Report (1999) looking at the failures of the Metropolitan Police while investigating the murder of Black student Stephen Lawrence. It is in this report that a very useful definition of institutional racism can be found:

Racism can exist in the following forms:

Prejudice – having a negative attitude about someone from another 'race' or ethnic group.

Discrimination – acting in a way that treats people from another 'race' or ethnic group unequally.

Institutional racism – the intentional or unintentional actions of a public or private body that result in people from ethnic minority backgrounds being discriminated against.

The collective failure of an organisation to provide an appropriate and professional service to people because of their colour, culture or ethnic origin. It can be seen in processes, attitudes and behaviour which amount to discrimination through unwitting prejudice, ignorance, thoughtlessness and racist stereotyping which disadvantage minority ethnic people. (MacPherson 1999)

It is not just in the police force that institutional racism is evident. In section 7.3 of this chapter we will look at how prejudice and racist stereotyping within health and medical services adversely affect the health of ethnic minority people. Health professionals within the NHS also face institutional racism, with a variety of reports suggesting that health professionals from ethnic minority groups are worse off than White health professionals with equivalent training and expertise. This can range from unequal pay between White and minority doctors; barriers in going to medical school; or South Asian doctors being over-represented in junior grades and unpopular specialities. Overall, as Coker (2001) points out, this represents a regrettable loss of skill and talent for the NHS.

Question

What are your views on the levels of racism in society today? What do you think are the main issues and problems that we face in trying to bring about a more tolerant society?

7.3 Ethnicity, health and society

After looking at a great deal of information on what we mean by ethnicity, and some of its problems, plus levels and forms of racism, let us now see how all of this can affect the health of ethnic minority groups. Here, we shall look at class, the effects of racism and the negative experiences that ethnic minority groups can have of medical and health services. What is important to bear in mind here is that all the following are not discrete 'either/or' influences, but that they can work together simultaneously. Indeed, there is considerable overlap between all three issues. Racism pervades both class and experiences of care. One of the reasons why so many ethnic minority people are located in lower social classes is, in part, the experience of racism during migration to the UK from the 1950s onwards. Often ethnic groups encountered discrimination that prevented them from occupying better-paid jobs. Racism is also apparent in experiences of health and medical care, where, both intentional and unintentional, prejudice and discrimination affect how staff perceive, and react to, ethnic minority patients.

Class

Links

See Chapter 6 for more information on class and health.

As discussed in the introduction to this section on inequalities there is considerable overlap between all three inequalities of gender, ethnicity and class. They quite often interact to produce multiple problems for many people, resulting in their health being adversely affected. This is very true for many ethnic groups where class, and the effects of social deprivation, are also of great importance. Much research in the past has ignored, or underplayed, the role that class has in the health of ethnic groups. Recently though, some new research has sought to address that absence in our understanding of how ethnicity and class interact.

A great deal of evidence indicates that many ethnic minority groups in the UK experience social deprivation. Smaje (1995) and Karlsen et al. (2002) identified that many ethnic groups often live in socially deprived areas. Statistics (see Table 7.3 and 7.4 below) on poverty routinely indicate that ethnic minority groups experience greater levels of poverty and unemployment than the majority White group in the UK.

From the evidence presented above, and by keeping in mind the material in Chapter 6 that deals with class and health, it appears that class should influence the health of ethnic minority groups. As we shall see, this is very much the case but as Nazroo (1998) warns, ethnicity should not be reduced to class. This means that we should just not think that we can drop ethnicity as a reason for people's poor health and claim that it is all down to class; we should see both as having very real and damaging effects. What the research reveals is that people from an ethnic minority group can be in the same class as people from the White majority group, but will be further disadvantaged, and be located towards the lower end of that particular class. So, we find, for example, that White people in the Registrar-General's classes IV and V have low mean weekly incomes, but people from Indian or African Asian, Caribbean, and – lowest of all – Pakistani or Bangladeshi, ethnic groups have even lower mean weekly incomes (Nazroo 2006). Ethnic minority groups are also more likely to have more insecure jobs, more unsocial hours, and worse housing than White people of the same

TABLE 7.3   *Economic activity, by ethnic group in the UK (SPIU 2002)*

	Economic Activity rate (ages 16–59/64)	Employment rate	ILO Unemp.rate all ages 16+
White	79.4	75.9	4.4
All ethnic minority groups	64.7	57.4	11.1
Mixed	70.0	62.2	11.1
Asian	61.9	55.4	10.6
Black	71.1	61.8	12.9
Chinese	58.3	54.1	–
Other ethnic groups	58.3	52.8	9.2

TABLE 7.4   *Percentage resident in area of deprivation by quintile and ethnic group (Nazroo 2006: 7)*

Townsend score	White	Caribbean	Indian	Pakistani & Bangladeshi
Highest quintile	20.4	3.3	5.8	1.0
	20.2	5.1	9.5	1.6
	20.1	11.3	9.9	4.0
	19.4	8.0	26.3	12.7
Lowest quintile	19.8	72.3	48.5	80.6

Reproduced by kind permission of Routledge

class. Class differences also exist within ethnic groups, ethnic minority people with non-manual occupations having better health over a range of indicators than those of the same ethnic group in manual occupations (see Table 7.5).

The experience of racism

There is a growing body of research which shows that the experience of racism has a debilitating effect on health. Karlsen and Nazroo (2002a, 2004) in the UK, Krieger et al. (2005) in the US and Harris et al. (2006) in New Zealand, for example, have all come to similar conclusions that we have to take the lived experience of racism seriously if we are to have a full and rounded understanding of what contributes to ethnic health inequalities. This racism can come in a variety of forms, whether the day-to-day racism of name-calling and prejudice; actual physical abuse and assault; or dealing with institutional racism. It is also important is that it is just not *direct* but also *indirect* experience of racism that that has an effect. This means that someone does not have to be name-called in the street or attacked: they simply need to have a perception that these things exist and that it could happen to them – in short, a fear of racism and the worry and stress this creates (Karlsen and Nazroo 2004). In many ways indirect experiences of racism share an affinity

TABLE 7.5   *Fair, poor, or very poor reported health compared with others of the same age by socio-economic position.*

	White[1]	Indian or African Asian[2]	Pakistani or Bangladeshi[3]	Caribbean[4]
Occupational class				
Non-manual	21.5	19.9	30.2	25.0
Manual	22.6	27.4	35.1	29.4
No full-time worker in household	36.7	33.9	44.1	38.2
Unweighted base	2110	1782	1592	1060
Tenure				
Owner-occupier	22.6	24.4	34.7	26.6
Tenant	34.5	33.7	45.0	40.0
Unweighted base	2173	1848	1692	1077

1 p < 0.01 for both occupational class and tenure
2 p < 0.01 for both occupational class and tenure
3 p < 0.01 for both occupational class and tenure
4 p < 0.01 for both occupational class and tenure

Source: Nazroo, James Y. (2001: 117) *Ethnicity, class and Health*. London: PSI (PSI report no. 880)
Reproduced with permission of the copyrignt holders, PSI

with the stress–related psycho–social pathways of health that we explored in Chapter 6 on class and health.

This stress created by racism is clearly seen in research by Chahal and Julienne (1999). What they noted was that for Black and ethnic minority people racism was an everyday experience. This could have quite far-reaching and long-term consequences in their private lives and affected how they interacted with friends, family and the wider community. For example, worrying about and feeling stressed by racism could mean feeling anxious about leaving one's home at night, or allowing the children to play outside. Mundane tasks could become fraught with danger. One woman in the study said that she found it difficult to put the washing out during the day as this could lead to her being abused by a neighbour. Overall, the people in this study felt tired, worn out, stressed, depressed, vulnerable and isolated by their experiences of racist victimisation.

Question

The above discussion points out that racism does not have to be directly experienced in the form of verbal abuse or assault, for instance, to have a negative impact on health; the idea that one could be subject to racism also has a similarly poor outcome for health. Why do you think this is so?

For ethnic minority people who have been either verbally abused or physically attacked the chances of assessing their health as poor are greatly increased. Karlsen and Nazroo (2002b) reported that those who were verbally abused were around 50 per cent more likely to see their health as poor but those who had direct experience had just over 100 per cent greater chance of reporting their health as being poor.

Negative experiences of medical and health care

Reviewing a range of research and reports, Chahal (2004) concluded that medical and health care services can be problematic for Black and ethnic minority people, with negative experiences of medical and health services being a common problem. This is particularly evident with mental health services. Black people are over-represented in mental illness statistics, more likely to be placed in secure wards and to receive different – if not poorer – treatment and care than Whites. As ever, research findings beg the question of why is this so. Delving a little deeper we can see a picture of intentional and unintentional prejudice, racism of various kinds and a general lack of cultural sensitivity. To answer the question in more detail we shall look at why there is over-representation of Black people in the statistics, how Black people come into contact with services and the treatment that is offered.

Pathways to care: ethnic minorities' initial contact with psychiatric services

One of the most common pathways for African-Caribbean people to come into contact with psychiatric services is via the police. From their research, Pilgrim and Rogers (1993) identified multiple interconnecting reasons. Black people, especially young Black men, are more likely to be regarded as potentially threatening and/or dangerous than White people. These attitudes exist not only among the public, for the Stephen Lawrence Inquiry found examples of institutionalised racism within the Metropolitan Police Force. Here we see the police, an important part of the 'control culture' in British society, reflecting and acting on the wider racist attitudes that exist in society. Therefore, when the police come into contact with young Black men they are more likely to react and interpret their behaviour in a negative manner. This negativity can extend to the judiciary. Pilgrim and Rogers also noted that Black people have a different perception of services from White users, whether one of mistrust or of cynicism about the quality of treatment they might receive.

Treatment

When people from Black or Asian communities are offered treatment, the form and quality of the services on offer can again be different from those offered to White service users. Reviewing the literature on treatment of ethnic minorities, Pilgrim and Rogers (1993: 57) noted that 'Black people are treated in a more coercive and punitive way within the psychiatric system'. They cited various examples of research which indicated that Black people, even when they were non-violent, tended to receive more medication over the period of their treatment and that medication was more likely to include major tranquillisers. In addition, African-Caribbean patients were more often seen as potentially threatening or aggressive.

Problems exist for Black and Asian people in aftercare and when living in the community. The ever-present problem of racism emerged clearly in Radia's (1996) study of Asians with mental health problems living in the four London boroughs of Brent, Harrow, Ealing and Tower Hamlets. Respondents here reported that they feared racial assault and abuse on the streets. Service provision was also noted to be poor and lacking in cultural sensitivity, with Asian people in this study often being subject to stereotyping by service providers. Common myths were that Asian people would be looked after 'by their own' and that services were not wanted because no one came forward. The lack of cultural sensitivity came through when conceptualising mental illness. Western notions of the mind and body being separate entities are not shared by Asian people, who see both existing as a whole. Fenton and Sadiq-Sangster (1996) have also noted this point. They found that south Asian women conceptualised mental distress using metaphors that shared images and expressions of mind and body. In their study feelings of being stressed and of low mood were expressed as 'thinking-too-much-in-the-heart'.

Links

See Chapter 9 for more information on mental health.

Other research has also noted a lack of cultural sensitivity within service provision. Researching counselling providers in Glasgow, Leeds, Bristol and London, Netto et al. (2001) reported that a lack of awareness of cultural and religious factors could have a negative impact on the uptake and success of counselling services for Asian and Black people. They suggested that services could be improved by increasing access to counselling for Black people; by increasing the number of trained counsellors with appropriate experience and/or training in cultural sensitivity; by reviewing service provision in order to obtain feedback from Black service users; and by encouraging the Black community to question their own attitudes to mental health to make it easier for Black people with mental health problems to come forward.

Irish people and mental health

So far, we have concentrated on the experiences of Black and Asian people but there exists another ethnic minority in the UK that also experiences difficulties. This minority has a distinct problem, namely invisibility, because until quite recently they were classified as part of the indigenous White population. Here we are referring to Irish-born people living in Britain. Even though Irish-born people may outwardly appear to share the characteristics of native-born White people in terms of skin colour and language there are many cultural subtleties that are overlooked by service providers and by society as a whole.

Irish-born people face the following problems:

- lack of services designed for Irish-born people;
- high unemployment;
- high levels of mental and physical health problems;
- reduction in life expectancy on immigration to England. (MIND 2000b)

Conclusion

Current research and sociological thinking on 'race', ethnicity and health is beginning to develop a much more subtle and nuanced appreciation of the way in which various factors and social structures influence the health of ethnic minority groups in society. What is becoming clearer is that, to begin with, we must be very careful about making sweeping generalisations about terms such as 'race' and ethnicity. Problems, stereotypes and, at worst, prejudices can often be bundled up in these concepts. For example, the concept of ethnicity can often depict a minority group as being culturally static, with other important divisions, such as class, being absent. As the evidence and research discussed in this chapter indicated, this can be far from the lived experiences of people in minority groups.

We also saw that the major cause of ethnicity and health inequalities is not to be found in the particular cultures of the people in minority groups, but in racism. The negative effects can be experienced either directly (name calling in the street) or indirectly (the anxiety created by anticipation of being subjected to some form of racism). This can also be present in the care provision, with people from ethnic minority groups sometimes encountering prejudice and/or inappropriate services.

This illustrates once more that it is powerful social forces that exist above and beyond the individual that shape and influence health, often more so than the choices and actions of individuals themselves.

SUMMARY POINTS

- There has been a Black presence in Britain for thousands of years.
- The non-White population of the UK is now 7.9 per cent.
- Increasing numbers of people are from mixed backgrounds.
- 'Race' lacks any scientific validity as a way of categorising and differentiating people. Genetically people the world over are virtually the same.
- The concept of 'race' is historically quite new and developed out of European colonialism and slavery.
- Racism can be a defining experience for many ethnic minority people.
- Ethnicity can be a more useful way of exploring different groups of people with its emphasis on the social and cultural aspects of people's lives. It too can be problematic at times. Sometimes ethnicity can be used to imply that culture is static and some ethnic classifications are too broad in their coverage.
- Class and socio-economic differences affect the health of ethnic minority groups.
- The health of ethnic minority people is often worse than the health of White people in the same class.
- Within the same ethnic minority group there are differences in health, with those from the non-manual occupation class having better health than those in manual occupation classes.
- The psycho-social effects of racism can have a strong impact on the health of ethnic minority groups.
- Ethnic minorities people can have negative experiences of health and medical services, encountering either inappropriate care or prejudice and discrimination.

Case study

Mike remembers what his dad told him about what he had to endure at work back in the 1970s. Being the first African-Caribbean person to work in the local council housing department he had to deal with all sorts of abuse and disrespect. Sometimes, this was out-and-out racism. A small group of people in the office often verbally abused him. On several occasions they left bananas or literature from far-right racist parties on his desk. What Mike's dad found worse though were the attitudes of other office workers, who, even though not openly hostile to him, always seemed a little suspicious. Mike's dad had to constantly make jokes about his skin colour in order to be accepted in any way. He hated having to act in that way as he found it demeaning. This added an extra layer of stress to an already stressful job. It was having to deal with all these issues that, Mike believes, led to his dad developing a heart condition in his late fifties. In fact, his dad had to take early retirement as a result of his poor health. To this day he still claims to feel quite poorly most of the time and not as healthy as he would like to be.

For Mike, many of these problems are firmly in the past. The office in which he works is like the rest of the city, with a mixed, cosmopolitan and diverse workforce. He works alongside people who are White, Asian or African-Caribbean, who, like him, see themselves as British born and bred. He gets on well with just about everyone in his section and he faces none of the outward racism that his dad had to face. However, the more subtle forms of racism persist. Mainly, this is to do with the management. Despite the diversity of the workforce, the management are uniformly White. He has put in for promotion several times but each time he has been rejected. This is even though he has worked hard, put in the hours and is respected by many of his colleagues as a good worker. Other people with a less strong profile than his have advanced up the ranks much quicker than him. He now suspects that it is something to do with his ethnicity. Regardless of how much he works, it just never seems enough. This is starting to get to him. Lately, he has found himself becoming more stressed and generally down.

1 What elements of the case study reflect some of the wider social changes that were discussed in this chapter?
2 Discuss the ways in which racism has had an effect on the health of both Mike today and his father in the past.
3 Besides issues to do with ethnicity, what other social factors could be exerting an influence on Mike's health?

Taking your studies further

This chapter will have helped you understand many of the key terms, concepts, theories and debates relating to 'race', ethnicity and health. Listed below are journal articles and books that will provide deeper and more detailed discussions of the points raised in this chapter. You will also find what is available on the companion website. This offers downloads of relevant material, plus links to useful websites in addition to podcasts and other features.

Recommended reading

Books

Nazroo, J. (2001) *Ethnicity, Class and Health*. London: PSI.
Nazroo, J. (ed.) (2006) *Health and Social Research in Multiethnic Societies*. London: Routledge.

Journal articles

Higginbottom, G.M.A. (2006) '"Pressure of life": ethnicity as a mediating factor in mid-life and older people's experience of high blood pressure', *Sociology of Health and Illness,* 28 (5): 583–610.

Karlsen, S. and Nazroo, J.Y. (2002) 'Agency and structure: the impact of ethnic identity and racism on the health of ethnic minority people', *Sociology of Health and Illness,* 24 (1): 1–20.

Karlsen, S. and Nazroo, J.Y. (2002) 'The relationship between racial discrimination, social class and health among ethnic minority groups', *American Journal of Public Health,* 92 (4): 624–31.

Karlsen, S. and Nazroo, J. (2004) 'Fear of racism and health', *Journal of Epidemiology and Community Health,* 58: 1017–18.

Krieger, N. (2003) 'Does racism harm health? Did child abuse exist before 1962? On explicit questions, critical science, and current controversies: an ecosocial perspective', *American Journal of Public Health,* 93 (2): 194–9.

Website

BBC online Race UK http://news.bbc.co.uk/hi/english/static/in_depth/uk/2002/race/

On the companion website

Fenton, S. and Charsley, K. (2000) 'Epidemiology and sociology as incommensurate games: accounts from the study of health and ethnicity', *Health,* 10 (4): 403–25.

Williams, S.J. (2003) *Medicine and the Body*. London: Sage. Chapter 2 on ''Structuring'' bodies: emotions, inequalities and health'.

companion website ↖

8

Gender and health

MAIN POINTS

- The sociological study of gender and health is in a period of change.
- 'New' perspectives are taking over from 'traditional' perspectives.
- Emphasis now lies on understanding the lived experiences of both women and men and acknowledging that differences exist within each sex.
- 'Traditional' explanations concerning early male mortality and excess female morbidity are under question.
- Gender relations are increasingly complex with many challenges to male dominance in society.
- Gender theories now emphasise the complexities of many varied forms of masculinities and femininities.
- Men, too, can suffer from ideas of what it is to be male and 'macho' in today's society.

KEY CONCEPTS

Gender, patriarchy, inequality, masculinities, femininities.

Introduction

The study of **gender** and health has recently undergone a period of change and transition. New and interesting ways of thinking about how being a woman or a man affects your health are currently being developed and debated. This is in contrast with more 'traditional' perspectives of discussing gender and health, where the main perspectives could be easily summarised as 'men die and women suffer'. This was due to much of medical sociology in the past (mainly from the 1970s) putting forward the view that, when it comes to health differences between men and women, men experience higher levels of earlier mortality, while women live longer but experience higher levels of morbidity during their lives. The reasons for these differences were often explained by reference to paid and domestic work roles, as well as the wider, and often stereotypical, social roles, which men and women held. Another important, if somewhat unintentional feature of 'traditional' perspectives on gender and health was that, more often than not, gender meant women and not women *and* men. This was probably due to the influence of **feminism** in this particular area of sociological research.

Though traditional perspectives on gender and health produced a great deal of vital and interesting research, recently certain sociologists, such as Kandrack et al. (1991), Annandale and Hunt (2000) and Macintyre et al (1999), have called for a rethink of how we both look at and understand gender and health. Much of this rethink has been prompted by two influences. Firstly, we live in a **society** of increasingly complex gender relations. Many of the old assumptions about gender – for instance the man as breadwinner, going out to earn the family wage and the woman staying at home tending to domestic chores – simply no longer fit today's society. There have been many other transformations, shifts and movements in how women and men relate to the home, to work and to each other. In the midst of all this change women's and men's health is affected in new ways. Secondly, there is growing questioning of the theories used to conceptualise gender. The main point of contention is that we need to adequately understand how issues relating to gender affect both sexes and must take on board the varied experiences of men and women.

In this chapter, we shall take a journey through the research, literature and sociological perspectives on gender and health and, in doing so, we will make several distinct stops on the way. We shall begin with a review of what sociologists mean by gender, pointing to how ideas of what it means to be a man or woman are not fixed but depend on the place or society where you are. This discussion will then expand on to some of the statistics that help us understand the situation of women and men today, before looking at some theoretical perspectives. We shall then look at how and where medical sociology finds itself, as it takes on the challenge of understanding gender and health in more complex times. Finally we shall look at how ideas of what it is to be masculine and feminine affect people's health.

8.1 Thinking about gender in contemporary society

Before we begin to look at wider issues of gender it is useful to define the two key terms of **sex** and gender. 'Sex' refers to the biological differences between men and women and how anatomical features lead to some being identified as male or female. On the other hand, 'gender' refers to the social, cultural and psychological aspects of being a woman or a man. Often the two terms are used interchangeably in some research and writing about women and men. In the rest of this chapter, we shall be quite strict in their usage and the definitions just given will be adhered to.

Let us now consider and think about what we mean by gender. For many people that will seem a rather obvious question to answer, with gender being decided by the biological body that we have. This line of thought also assumes that the types of behaviour that men and women engage in are decided by biology. Sociologists, however, have argued strongly that the answer is nowhere near as clear-cut as that. By comparing cultures in different places and across times we find that what constitutes being a man or a woman is *extremely variable*. All sorts of examples can be used to illustrate this. For instance, among the Wodaabe tribe, who live in the African country of Niger, it is the men who wear the make-up and act in what to western eyes would be a feminine manner.

Equally interesting examples can be found in the industrialised west. One gender stereotype, for instance, is that women are not suited to heavy industrial work and should not be employed in hazardous factories, but would be more appropriately employed as secretaries in safe office environments. During the Second World War the requirements of fighting the war turned that stereotype on its head. With many men away fighting at the front, there were few men left to do the heavy industrial work such as building aircraft or making munitions, which were vital for the war effort. As a consequence government-backed drives, both in the USA and UK, attempted to get women into the factory to do that vital war work. In America, 'Rosie the Riveter' (see Image 8.1) spearheaded one campaign to attract women into the workplace. What's interesting about the image of Rosie is her depiction as being 'feminine', with headscarf and make-up, while at the same time displaying the very 'masculine' traits of the strong muscular arm and the factory overalls. The poster's tag-line, 'We Can Do it!' is a very assertive statement about the capabilities of

Gender, refers to the social, cultural and psychological differences between men and women. **Sex** refers to the biological differences between men and women.

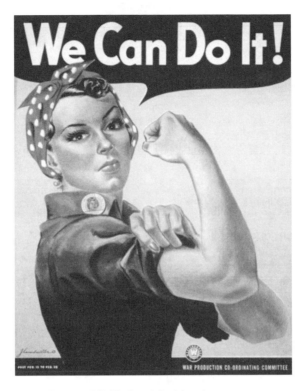

IMAGE 8.1   *Rosie the Riveter (US National Archives)*
Image courtesy of US National Archives

women. At the height of the war approximately 30 per cent of all working women in the US were in factories, with employers in 1942 increasing the number of jobs that they thought suitable for women from 29 per cent to 55 per cent of all occupations (Colman 1995). After the war this role-reversal was not to continue, however, with women on both sides of the Atlantic being encouraged to leave the factory jobs that they had occupied during the war and to make the return to the domestic sphere.

What the example of 'Rosie the Riveter' tells us is that what it means to be a man or a woman is not a fixed entity but is frequently defined by the needs and attitudes of a society at a given time. When American and British society needed female workers to meet shortages in the arms industry attitudes changed to allow for that to happen, and when women were no longer required to fill those posts then attitudes changed again. It is not just society, or the needs of industry in the above example, which influences what it means to be a man or a woman. In the 1960s and 1970s, throughout Europe and North America, the rise of the Women's Movement saw the self-organisation of feminist women directly challenge prevailing social norms of

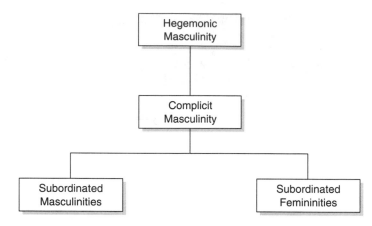

FIGURE 8.1   *Connell's gender hierarchy*

what a woman's place in society should be. The old notions that the woman belonged passively in the home, looking after her husband and children were brought into question, with women at this time fighting for and adopting more active roles, whether in the workplace or in their private lives. Indeed, many of the job opportunities and increased control over their lives experienced by women today is attributable to the success of the struggles of the sixties and seventies.

Question

The above discussion looks at what it is to be a man or a woman. What do you think are masculine or feminine characteristics today? Do you see any changes in how men or women relate to each other in everyday life?

Theorising gender

Within **sociology** of health and illness how we theorise gender has shifted away from 'out-and-out' feminist theories, which concentrated on how women are dominated by men, to theories that focus on gender relations and gender order. These theories look at how interactions between men and women are affected by the ideas of masculinity and femininity that pervade society (Annandale and Hunt 2000). This is not to claim that we should drop all the insights that feminist theories gave us nor to suggest, for one moment, that we have moved away from a society where gender ceases to act as an arbiter of power and privilege, particularly in favour of men. For instance, feminist theories, which provided a rich **analysis** of **patriarchy** (male domination), allowed us to understand how society on a variety of fronts privileges men. This, though, does not take into account the experiences of men and implies that all men are part of a 'unified' bloc, who all share similar dispositions, access to power and economic resources, for example. Current theoretical thinking on gender acknowledges that there exist many varieties of 'maleness' and masculinity in society (as well as 'femaleness' and femininity), which should also be acknowledged and theorised. Whitehead (2002: 16) usefully summarises the many different expressions of masculinities that exist in the world today:

> … from the 'gym queens' to suited politicians, from Boy George to Arnold Schwarzenegger, from the ageing leathered 'biker' to the ageing hippy 'drop-out'. From the gun-toting LA (or Manchester) gang member to the male nurse, from Rupert Murdoch to the black 'rapper', from 'Masters of the Universe' to the male charity worker, from the Muslim cleric to the atheist househusband, from Mike Tyson to Danny Glover, indeed from profeminist man to the Christian 'promise keepers'…"

Connell (2005) has provided a highly insightful **theory** of gender that brings an understanding of masculinity and patriarchy into an overall theory of gender relations and gender order. Central to his ideas is that we cannot understand masculinity and femininity unless we see them as related to and shaping each other. This relationship, however, is not equal and, by and large, it is men who continue to be dominant in society. This power is played out in the day-to-day interactions between men and women in their private and public lives and is informed by wider societal ideas of what it is to be masculine and feminine.

There exists, for Connell, a gender order in western capitalist societies (see Figure 8.1). At the top, and the most powerful element, of this gender order is **hegemonic masculinity**, to which all other forms of masculinity and femininity are subordinate. The concept refers to how one form of masculinity (in this case one which is healthy, heterosexual, wealthy, assertive, aggressive and white) is associated with power, being successful and being the form of masculinity that should be aspired to in western societies. By being the 'top dog', so to speak, this form of masculinity is hegemonic, which means it controls everything else. Some good examples of men who epitomise hegemonic masculinity are the British motor-car TV presenter Jeremy Clarkson, and in America, the former actor and now governor of California, Arnold Schwarzenegger. Next in the gender order is *complicit masculinity*. This is a form of masculinity that may not live up to the full expectations of hegemonic masculinity, but still affords a reasonable amount of power. We then see subordinated masculinities and femininities which are beneath both hegemonic and complicit masculinity in terms of power and status. *Subordinated masculinities* include gay men, and in terms of health, men whose masculinity is challenged or undermined

Patriarchy refers to male domination in society and can be expressed both privately and publicly in culture, economic, politics and through physical violence. **Matriarchy** refers to a society that is female dominated. See chapter 1 for more on feminist theory.

Hegemonic masculinity refers to the dominant form of masculinity in society. Currently, this would refer to men who are healthy, wealthy, white and powerful and act in a 'macho' manner. Very few men live up to this expectation but it exerts a strong influence over both men and women.

by physical and mental illness. *Subordinated femininities* include *emphasised femininity*, which refers to women who comply with hegemonic masculinity, and this involves matching up to hegemonic male expectations of attractiveness and femininity. In terms of health, this can mean, especially for older women, taking on care duties for children, disabled people or older relatives in the home. There also exists *resistant femininity* where women reject the demands and norms of emphasised femininity. This tends to be a less visible group of women (for example, lesbians and spinsters) in society, given the prevalence and profile of emphasised femininity.

Gender relations today

A key theme throughout this chapter has been the increasing complexity of the many aspects of gender in contemporary society whether this is to do with work, relationships or the home. In short, what we see today is that the deeper constraints on women (such as their sole focus in life being the home) are very much weaker, with women experiencing much more control and choice in their working and personal lives in comparison with previous generations of women. Parallel to the strengthening of women in society we see a weakening of male dominance in a variety of fields. For example, there have been changes in the economy, where the traditional male heavy manufacturing industries are giving way to female-dominated service industries. This is leading to a feminisation of the workforce.

This, though, should *not* be taken to mean that we now see complete equality of the sexes. Overall, there are many signs of equality in some areas but that has to be set against many other signs that things have not changed that much for women. If we look at some examples, this will become clearer. In terms of employment, we find that in the UK in 2005 each sex carried out 13.3 million jobs – roughly a fifty-fifty split of all jobs. On the surface this is a major shift, since in 1985 men performed 2 million more jobs than women (ONS 2006). If we delve a little deeper we find inconsistencies. Even though there is strong female participation in the workforce (see Figure 8.2), the majority of those women will employed part-time.

Another interesting complexity can be seen in the types of occupation in which women and men are located, and the disparities in their pay. What we see here is a picture of women making gains in some occupations but none in others. If we look at Figure 8.3, we can see some of these trends. For example, there is increasing parity of women and men in middle-class professions and associated professions, with women also making gains in management. This, though, should be contrasted with more working-class occupations. Here we see a familiar pattern of men occupying the skilled trades and women in secretarial and administration.

If we turn now to the income gap between women and men we can see it beginning to close. Figure 8.4 indicates that women are catching up with men. However,

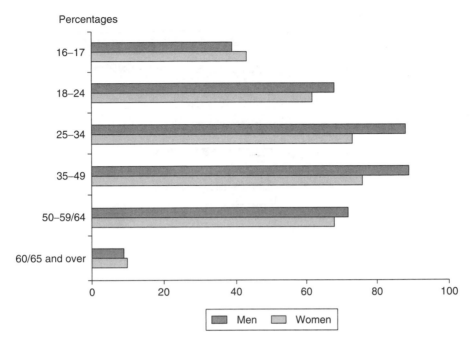

FIGURE 8.2   *Participation in the workforce by age and sex (ONS 2004)*
Source: National Statistics website: www.statistics.gov.uk
Crown copyright material is reproduced with the permission of the Controller of HMSO
Reproduced under the terms of the Click-Use Licence

according to the Fawcett Society, it will still take another eighty-five years for women to completely catch up with men (Hall 2003)!

8.2 Understanding gender and health – at a crossroads?

Annandale and Hunt (2000) have recently pointed out that research in the study of gender and health is at a crossroads with 'traditional' approaches giving way to 'new' approaches. Put simply, the 'traditional' approaches often (though unintentionally) put forward the view that men and women were located in very distinct and different social roles (notably, men in full-time paid work and women in the home). These social roles required them to act in certain ways, which were, generally speaking, good for men but bad for women. The 'new' approaches hold that social roles may be

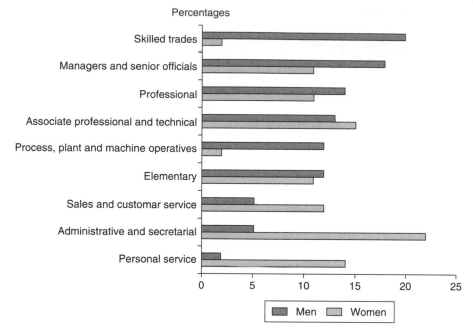

FIGURE 8.3   *Participation of women in selected occupations by sex (ONS 2004)*
Source: National Statistics website: www.statistics.gov.uk
Crown copyright material is reproduced with the permission of the Controller of HMSO
Reproduced under the terms of the Click-Use Licence

According to Annandale and Hunt (2000) we can identify 'traditional' and 'new' perspectives on gender and health. 'Traditional' perspectives focus mainly on seeing *differences* between women and men, and focus on excess early male mortality and higher female morbidity. 'New' perspectives focus on seeing the *differences* and *similarities* both between and within women and men, and acknowledge the increasing complexity of gender relations in contemporary society.

'masculine' or 'feminine' in orientation (such as running a business or looking after children) but a man may carry out a 'feminine' role (looking after the children), while a woman may occupy a 'masculine' role (running a business). The 'new' approaches also focus on how men and women experience those roles and how those experiences affect their health (Annandale and Hunt 2000). The more 'feminine' a role, the lower status it tends to have and this can lead to poor health. Performing feminine roles also carries much more pressure than performing male roles.

Annandale and Hunt (2000: 27–9) usefully summarise the differences between what they see as 'traditional' and 'new' approaches to gender and health:

- 'Traditional' forms of research had the tacit assumption that what was good for men was bad for women when it came to health. 'New' research follows a more nuanced and subtle approach, and understands that similar circumstances may have *similar* or *different* consequences for the health of men and women.

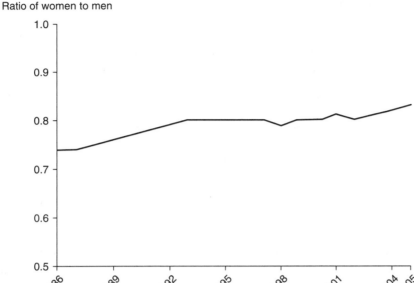

FIGURE 8.4   *Income ratio of women to men over time. (ONS 2004)*
Source: National Statistics website: www.statistics.gov.uk
Crown copyright material is reproduced with the permission of the Controller of HMSO
Reproduced under the terms of the Click-Use Licence

- 'New' approaches are aware of the differences *within* men and *within* women. In 'traditional' research men, in particular, were treated as an undifferentiated group, where all men had similar health experiences.
- In 'traditional' research positivist, quantitative, statistical methods were predominant. In 'new' research the role of qualitative method is highlighted in trying to obtain an understanding of how the experiences of men and women shape their health. This does not mean abandoning quantitative approaches but understanding that alone they do not provide a full picture of gender and health.

We shall now look at some 'new' thinking on morbidity and mortality rates for women. In the introduction we looked at how much 'traditional' research and thinking made the observation that 'men die early and women spend more of their lives unwell'. The 'new' thinking challenges some of these assumptions as to what causes these differences.

Gender and morbidity

One long-held view (for example, Hibbard and Pope 1986) is that women have higher morbidity rates than men. There have been different attempts to explain this over the years, for example:

- Women do experience more ill-health than men because of the demands of their social roles.
- Women are more disposed to seek help than men.
- Women are more 'in-tune' with their bodies.
- Surgeries are not male friendly and put men off seeking help.
- It is easier for women to adopt the sick role.

There may be something in the above explanations. Indeed, in Chapter 9 on mental health we see how attachment to, and experience of, certain roles can result in other levels of distress for women. However, if we turn to the statistical evidence, on which the assumptions of higher female morbidity are often based, Macintyre et al. (1996, 1999) have raised a few concerns. They argue that on closer inspection of the evidence the actual picture of gender morbidity is very complex, and is very much dependent on where a woman or a man is in their **life cycle** and which particular type of illness you are considering. So, for example, younger males tend to report more long-standing and limiting illness than females. When it comes to type of illness we see a great variety and no clear pattern. Macintyre et al. (1996) also report no real sex difference for men and women of any age currently experiencing conditions such as diabetes, respiratory disorders or epilepsy.

Gender and mortality

Following on from the points raised above concerning morbidity, another long-standing perception, when looking at gender and health, is that women have some form of biological advantage in terms of life expectancy. In the UK, for instance, a female born in 2004 can expect to live until she is 81.1 years old, while a male born in the same year can expect to reach the age of 76.7 years (ONS 2006). Such statistics strongly suggest that women do enjoy some form of biological advantage over men, but, again, we must exercise caution before making any firm statements. Mick Carpenter (2000: 49) makes several important points about always seeking to find differences between men and women when, in fact, there are more similarities in the life and health experiences of women and men. He notes that the life expectancy of both men and women has improved significantly since the 1800s (see Figure 8.5). Indeed, the gap between men and women appears to be closing, with men increasingly catching up with women as we enter the twenty-first century.

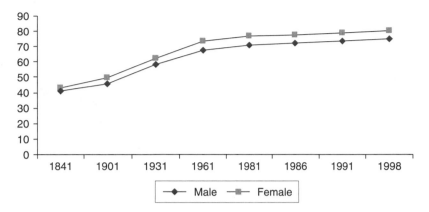

FIGURE 8.5 *Changes in male and female mortality, 1840–1998. (ONS 2006b)*
Source: National Statistics website: www.statistics.gov.uk
Crown copyright material is reproduced with the permission of the Controller of HMSO
Reproduced under the terms of the Click-Use Licence

We should also consider that the sizeable life expectancy advantage that women experience in the UK is very much a western phenomenon. If we look at Figure 8.6, we can see that overall women do have longer lives than men in most countries but this is extremely variable. On one hand, in some countries, such as Malawi, the life expectancy for both women and men is very low, while in Algeria there is a negligible difference in life expectancy for women and men. The reasons for this are multiple and diverse. For example, it depends on levels of health care a country can offer, where childbirth is safer, the levels of poverty and endemic illness, such as in Malawi, which faces widespread poverty and has many people infected with HIV/AIDS.

Bringing in men's health

One of the important shifts in the study of gender and health has been to acknowledge men and their experiences of health. It is, in some ways, ironic that the earlier research on gender and health focussed almost exclusively on women with little attention on men and their health. There have been calls by Banks (2001) and Doyal (2001), for example, for men's health to be more fully explored (see Box 8.1 for a summary). In the past, male health was held to be unproblematic, perhaps even the norm, and men benefited from hegemonic masculinity. It is becoming clear that this is not the case. Men, too, experience distinct health problems and they themselves can suffer as a result from the expectations of, and challenges to, masculinity in contemporary society. In the UK, for example, there is strong pressure for young men to live up to a 'laddish' lifestyle,

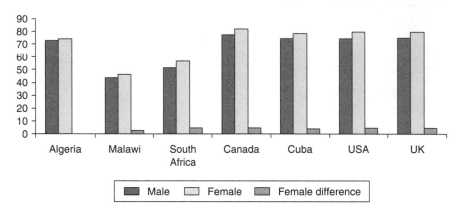

FIGURE 8.6   *Life expectancy by sex and selected country, 2002 (United Nations 2005)*

which involves demonstrating one's masculinity by engaging in potentially harmful and risky behaviours such as heavy drinking and driving fast cars. Indeed, many of the so-called 'lads' mags' are, arguably, replete with articles that extol such behaviour. The magazine *Nuts* (aimed at young men in their late teens), for instance, used to run a feature called 'Mate in a State', where readers were invited to send in photographs of their friends in highly inebriated states and caught in potentially compromising situations. The mortality and morbidity statistics show that one of the main causes of early death and injury for young men is alcohol related.

Box 8.1.   Williams (2003: 60–1) summarises the main reasons for an increasing interest in men's health:

- men do care about health issues but find it difficult to express their fears
- socially constructed gender characteristics (in addition to biological risk factors) are important in shaping the capacity of men and women to realize their full health potential
- men face particular problems because of the relation between masculine identity and risk taking
- greater sensitivity to sex and gender is needed in medical research, service delivery and wider social policies, including medical school training and consultations between male doctors and patients.

Masculinities and health

One of the emerging themes in the research that looks at male health is how individual men relate to dominant forms of (hegemonic) masculinity and how that affects their health and frames their experiences of illness (Watson 2000). Here, we shall look at some examples of this relationship and how it better informs us about men and their health.

As we saw earlier, the traditional research on gender and health drew attention to greater levels of morbidity for women. Though much recent thinking casts doubt on many of these explanations, work by O'Brien et al. (2005) indicates the complexities that exist in how men seek help, and how ideas of masculinity influence their decisions. In their study they conducted fourteen focus groups with men from a variety of backgrounds. The majority of the men, they found, preferred to be quite stoical in the face of illness and put off as long as possible seeking a consultation. Masculine ideas of being able to cope in the face of adversity, being able to endure pain and suffering, and not appearing to be weak or a 'sissy' were often voiced as reasons for keeping quiet about ill-health.

There were, however, some interesting exceptions to the 'keeping-it-to-yourself' attitudes expressed above. Men such as the firemen in the study – whose occupations gave them access to a very powerful masculine identity – indicated no real problems in communicating their health needs.

Overall, mental illness came to the fore as the one condition where greater reticence was reported in seeking help for fear of being seen to be unmanly. In fact, admitting to mental illness appeared to be the one area that offered the most direct challenge to masculinity. However, Emslie et al. (2006) in their research found that there were examples of some men who would talk about mental illness, in this case depression. Those that did either employed very masculine imagery of seeing their illness as part of a heroic struggle, or were aware that experiencing depression had allowed them to acknowledge a 'feminine' vulnerability as part of their identity.

Links

See Chapter 9 for more on how gender issues affect mental health, both for men and women.

Conclusion

Complexity and change is a motif throughout this chapter, both in terms of gender relations in society and what sociology has to say about how those gender relations are reflected in the health of women and men. The 'traditional' aphorism of 'men die, women suffer' that has been the dominant way of explaining gender inequalities has been demonstrated to be increasingly unhelpful. There are probably two factors at play here. First, many of the general gender inequalities to do with pay and employment, for example, that played a part in the poorer morbidity of women are beginning to be addressed and certain positive shifts towards some form of equality are discernible. This, though, should be tempered and placed firmly in perspective: while this progress is welcome (if not long overdue) and significant, there is still *much* to be done to bring about full equality.

Second, there has been a reconsideration of gender as a theoretical concept. A more nuanced approach is now visible in much of the research. The work of Connell has been highly noticeable. Men are being disaggregated from a homogeneous bloc and different ways of being male, and their attendant status, have been identified. This allows insights into how the roles and the actions of both men *and* women affect their health.

SUMMARY POINTS

- Gender is not fixed, but heavily influenced by society.
- Gender relations are becoming increasingly complex, with women making gains in some areas but not in others.
- In theorising gender it can be more effective to think of the power differences between different expressions of masculinity and femininity.

Case study

The following extract is from research by O'Brien, et al. (2005: 508). As mentioned earlier, this piece of research helps us understand further how masculinity influences men's decisions about seeking help for ill-health. Read the extract and then consider the questions below.

Rory: I broke my thumb and it took me two days before I went to see a doctor. … It was going septic, going green and purple and black and I was like 'I'm not going to bother them'.

Jake: I think that's a male trait.

Nathan:	Aye it's (*puts on a very deep voice*) 'I am man the hunter'. I think it's that.
Rory	I don't think it's that. ... It's just I couldnae go to the doctor's with that.
Nathan:	If a woman cut themselves they'd be away to the doctor. A guy'd be like 'I'll just go and get myself a bit of Sellotape and wrap it up'.
Rory:	Aye. I put a bit of tape on it and carried on.
Nathan:	That's just a man thing though isn't it?
Rory:	Aye that's just a man thing. 'I'm hard, I'm daft, I'll cut my arm off and just grow another one back.'

1 First of all, outline what is meant by 'hegemonic masculinity' and note down the names of men who exemplify such an expression of manhood.
2 In what ways are the men above influenced by prevailing ideas of masculinity?
3 By adhering to such ideas of masculinity how could it be damaging for their health?
4 How do you think these same young men would talk about mental health issues?
5 What could be done to assist men in discussing their health?

Taking your studies further

This chapter will have helped you understand many of the key terms, concepts, theories and debates relating to gender and health. Listed below are journal articles and books that will provide deeper and more detailed discussions of the points raised in this chapter. You will also find what is available on the companion website. This offers downloads of relevant material, plus links to useful websites in addition to podcasts and other features.

Recommended reading

Books

Annandale, H. and Hunt. K. (eds) (2000) *Gender Inequalities in Health.* Buckingham: Open University Press.

Journal articles

Courtenay, W.H. (2000) 'Constructions of masculinity and their influence on men's well-being: a theory of gender and health,' *Social Science and Medicine,* 50 (10): 1385–401.

Green, S.E. (2006) 'We're tired, not sad': benefits and burdens of mothering a child with a disability,' '"*Social Science and Medicine,* doi:10.1016/j.scomed2006.08.025.

O'Brien, R., Hunt, K. and Hart, G. (2005) 'It's caveman stuff, but that is to a certain extent how guys still operate,"' *Social Science and Medicine,* 61 (3): 503–16.

Watson, J. (2000) *Male Bodies: Health, Culture and Identity.* Buckingham: Open University Press.

Williams, C. (2000) `Doing health, doing gender: teenagers, diabetes and asthma,'. *Social Science and Medicine,* 50 (3): 387–96.

On the companion website

White, R. (2002) 'Social and political aspects of men's health,'. *Health,* 7 (6): 267–85.

Williams, S.J. (2003) *Medicine and the Body.* London: Sage. Chapter 2 on "Structuring" bodies: emotions, inequalities and health'.

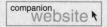

9

Mental health

MAIN POINTS

- Many more people in contemporary society are reporting and experiencing distress and depression
- Sociology helps us understand how mental health is framed in and by society.
- The attitudes of others and wider society greatly affect the well-being of those experiencing distress.
- Wider social inequalities are also visible in the distribution of diagnosed and reported mental health problems.

KEY CONCEPTS

Mental health, stigma, attitudes, class, gender, ethnicity, suicide.

Introduction

In 2006 'The Depression Report' made some very important and telling points about the extent of mental health problems in the United Kingdom. Not only did the report state that of all causes of disability, whether physical or mental, 40 per cent were accounted for by mental illness, but it found that tens of thousands of therapists were required to provide the necessary level of service to treat and assist the thousands of people who experience distress (LSE 2006). This report represents part of a trend within official policy circles and among the general population to treat mental illness as a serious issue. Throughout time, it has been regarded with suspicion and, sometimes, fear within **society** and seen as a lower-status field in which to practise by the medical profession. Much of this is to do with how social attitudes negatively frame mental illness. In previous centuries, for example, mental illness was seen as possession by demons, a curse by God. Even in more enlightened times it was the ultimate transgression against reason and rationality. As a result mental illness became stigmatised, the badge of the outsider and the deviant, associated with danger and violence.

Sociology has an important role to play in trying to understand the full intricacies of mental illness, especially when it comes to the ways in which society *influences* and *frames* both how we see mental health and illness and how society creates situations that can negatively impact on individual's mental health. Busfield (2000a: 554) neatly summarises what sociology can offer the study of mental health and illness, and how sociology tells us about:

> the importance of social processes in a range of areas: in the definition, boundaries and categories of mental disorder; in any adequate understanding of the factors that give rise to mental disorder; and in the understanding of the character of mental health practice and the professionals and others who shape that practice together with the ideas that underpin it.

This chapter will explore many of the issues associated with mental health and illness. Much of the focus, as suggested above, will be on how mental health and illness is framed by society. A great deal of the research indicates that this framing (attitudes held by the general public, how people's behaviour is interpreted by others, and the influence of medical classifications and categories) can affect the lives of people with mental health problems much more than the symptoms of their particular condition. We will look at some of the debates that exist in relation to defining and identifying what is seen to be mental illness. Attention will also be given to the effect that social attitudes, whether expressed by official bodies or by the lay general public, have on people who are experiencing some form of distress. This will lead us to the theory of **stigma**, which helps us understand how people with certain traits and characteristics are made to feel unwelcome and excluded by society. We will also look at depression in some depth. This will allow us to consider some of the particular circumstances and issues that affect people who experience this condition. Finally, consideration will be given to sociological perspectives on suicide.

9.1 What causes mental illness?

Giving a clear and concise answer to the question 'What causes mental illness?' is highly problematic. Part of the reason for this are the complexities and uncertainties that surround the whole process of diagnosis and identifying mental illness in the first place. Unlike physical illnesses, there is often no clear-cut objective sign that someone is experiencing a mental illness. One cannot, for example, find a broken bone or a cell that has become cancerous. Instead, doctors and psychiatrists have to rely on what people tell them; which is, in itself, highly problematic, as we shall see. McPherson and Armstrong (2006: 50) summarise these concerns well, when they say:

> What is pneumonia or appendicitis or cancer can be agreed internationally with reference to the presence or absence of certain clearly defined physical characteristics. In psychiatry, however, there is no such external biological referent to act as an anchor for diagnosis. Essentially, psychiatry classifies on the basis of a patient's patterns of symptoms which might vary according to how they are elicited and interpreted.

Because, then, we cannot always clearly identify what mental illness is, this makes the search for a cause all the harder. Lack of certainty means that no single authoritative answer can be put forward and we have seen over the years many competing explanations come and go. Broadly speaking, explanations for mental illness fall into one of two camps: biological explanations and social explanations. These look in very different directions and see quite different reasons for the existence of mental illness, as outlined below.

Even though there are often no apparent organic signs, biological explanations (often favoured by mainstream medicine) still privilege a focus on faulty genes or imbalances in the chemistry of the brain. There is, for instance, an association between low levels of serotonin and depression. This way of thinking, of looking for a biological cause, is increasingly reinforced by the proliferation of pharmaceutical interventions such as SSRIs (selective serotonin reuptake inhibitors) for treating depression, which suggest that if an illness can be treated by chemicals, then it must have a biological, organic basis.

Social explanations, on the other hand, fall into two general categories: social causation and social constructionist. The social causation perspective refers to how the various inequalities in society (mainly to do with **ethnicity**, **gender** and **class**) produce toxic levels of stress for some people. As a result of this stress, people may be 'tipped' into mental illness, whether it is a woman expected to bring up children on her own and keep down a job; or the experience someone from an ethnic minority group has of being racially abused by a neighbour; or the constant soul-destroying grind of poverty and not being able to lead the life that others enjoy. We shall look at some of these issues later, in sections 9.4 and 9.5.

The other main social explanation is social constructionist. Mental illness, from this viewpoint, is something that does not exist as a 'fact' or something that is 'real' and has absolutely no organic basis. This sociological view is influenced by the work of Foucault, who has argued that there is no single incontestable truth that can be discovered and agreed on by everyone. Rather, society is constructed by the ideas and conceputalisations of both individual people and also, more importantly, certain powerful groups. Some groups, such as psychiatrists, are able to construct a **discourse** that privileges a certain viewpoint above others, which allows them to effectively rule out and rule in ways of conceptualising, for example, what constitutes mental illness. Constructing such discourses allows such groups to become dominant in society and allows them to regulate and control the activities of others.

Links

See Chapter 1 for more information about Foucault and discourse.

Such a perspective allows us to question the factual basis of what is deemed to constitute mental illness, which is useful given the sometimes lack of solid evidence by which psychiatry proceeds. It also points to the way in which, as with other aspects, medicine can discipline and gain control over our lives.

Both biological and social explanations can definitely tell us something about mental illness. We have however, to be careful here of not falling into the trap that either explanation on its own is sufficient to address the complexity of mental health and illness. What is certain is that mental illness does not fit into simple

'A-leads-to-B-leads-to-C' type explanations. Rather, there is a complex interweaving of both society and biology, where both have to be understood as often working together in complex and dynamic ways.

Some of this complexity and dynamism in captured by Rose (2005) in his discussion of the causes of mental illness and how biology and society interact. He points out that just because a change in the chemistry of the brain takes place does not mean that the chemical change caused the illness. He urges that we must be careful in thinking about the processes which cause changes to happen. The example he uses to illustrate this point is that if someone has a headache, they take an aspirin. If we were then to check the chemicals in the person's brain in order to discover the chemical basis of a headache, we would find aspirin. Thus, according to the biological explanation, we would claim that aspirin causes headaches, because people who do not have headaches do not have the chemical aspirin present in their brains. Now, obviously, we know this not to be the case. What Rose is saying here is that, yes, chemical changes do occur, but they could equally be the *result* of other (in this case *social*) factors.

This takes us to an explanation put forward by Pilgrim and Rogers (1994), which acknowledges and develops that last point. They put forward a critical realist perspective on mental health and illness. This approach is useful in that it does not fall for the either/or impasse outlined above. Rather it brings in the consideration that to fully understand what causes misery and suffering in the world we have to be aware of one of the complexities of human life: that humans are simultaneously organic biological *and* social beings. This perspective allows us to see both aspects of being human as important and that humans are not entirely reducible to either. What this means is that a critical realist perspective fully acknowledges the strong and influential role of culture, but does not say that it is all down to society. It also accepts the importance of medical information and research, but, crucially, questions how diagnoses are framed by the social influences on the medical profession (this is explored further in the next section). Finally, a critical realist perspective accepts that biological processes are at work but, like Rose (2005) above, attempts to place those processes in a wider context where social factors may be the cause of biological changes.

Links

Chapter 1, section 1.2, provides an overview of sociological theories and perspectives.

9.2 Attitudes and constructions of mental health and illness

We usually accept medical terminology and classifications as given, that is, as being fact, value-free and scientific. Various sociologists and other writers, however, have challenged these notions. This is because medicine (like every other aspect of human activity) takes place within a social context. This social context influences in all sorts of subtle and not so subtle ways how people think. Those that work in medicine, such as doctors and psychiatrists, can also be quite easily influenced by, and in turn play an important role in, prevailing social attitudes. It is useful to remember this when thinking about mental illness and the way it is framed in and by society, especially when someone is judged to be acting in an 'unusual' and 'problematic' manner, for those judgements, made by doctors and psychiatrists, may be based not on purely neutral 'scientific' criteria but on social values and cultural norms (Foster 1995).

One useful example is the way in which both psychiatry and society have changed their perception of homosexuality. Until relatively recently, being gay was considered and framed as a form of mental illness. Gay men, for example, could find themselves on the receiving end of quite draconian interventions such as incarceration. During the 1960s, however, social attitudes towards homosexuality changed, partly due to the activities of campaign groups such as the Gay Liberation Front and events such as Stonewall when gay people fought back against police harassment. As the stigma and stereotyping diminished, so did the view that homosexuality was an illness rather than just one of the many forms of human sexuality.

Many myths and unhelpful images surround people deemed mentally ill. One common misconception is that people diagnosed with schizophrenia have a 'Jekyll and Hyde' personality, whereby they are sane and rational at one moment and violent and deranged the next (Angermeyer and Matschinger 1999). Unfortunately, these negative images appear to be widespread and persistent. Early research by Star (1955) identified negative stereotypes in the US, while similar work by Hall et al. (1993) in England found people possessing similar attitudes nearly forty years later and. Wider representations of mental illness also conflate and mix up mental illness and danger. More recently, Jorm, researching in Australia, has found that many members of the public have a very limited knowledge of mental illness. Using vignettes of someone with depression or schizophrenia Jorm found that few people could identify the depicted mental illness according to medical classifications: only 39 per cent correctly identified depression, and even less, 27 per cent, correctly identified schizophrenia Jorm (2000).

'Mental imbalance' often characterises many a movie or soap series villain. These are not just neutral images, however, that are contained within the safety of the cinema or the TV screen, but form beliefs and constructs held by people in everyday contexts. In turn these social stigmas increase the stress of those with mental illness and exacerbate feelings of social exclusion and social distance.

The 'Counting the cost' survey by Baker and MacPherson (2000) for MIND highlighted the extent of stigmatising images and the effects they had had on people with mental illness. For many respondents to the survey the social stigma was harder to deal with than the symptoms of their particular condition. Some key results from this survey are summarised below:

- 73 per cent of respondents felt that the media had been unfair, unbalanced or very negative over the previous three years.
- 12 per cent felt that the media had been fair, balanced or very positive.
- 50 per cent claimed that poor media coverage had a negative impact on their mental health.
- 24 per cent experienced some hostility from neighbours and their local communities as a result of media reports. (Baker and MacPherson 2000: 5)

Question

Why you think mental illness attracts such negative imagery?

Negative views of mental illness and mentally ill people are also evident among young people. The 'Tomorrow's Minds' survey reached a similar conclusion on stereotyping and **prejudice** (Baker and MacPherson 2000). Sixty per cent of young people in the survey admitted to using abusive terms such as 'psycho', 'schizo', 'nutter' or 'loony' to describe mentally ill people.

Historically, these images of mental illness have their roots in ideas of demonic possession (Scheff 1966) or the loss of rationality (Foucault 1967). Currently, negative images of mental illness are presented in newspaper articles, films, documentaries and popular dramas. Again, we see a dominance of stereotypes and misleading images. Philo (1996) noted that the majority of images were associated with violence, particularly violence towards other people, though also to self. The reasons for so many negative images being dominant in the media is not necessarily to do with the prejudiced attitudes of programme makers; rather, it is to do with the restraints imposed by the format of television shows, especially soaps. Programmes are restricted to half-hour slots, have multiple plot-lines and a need to provide dramatic entertainment that unfolds over a relatively short period of time. Realistic portrayals, therefore, of mental illness with all the various subtleties and intricacies that distressed individuals experience are ignored or glossed over. In addition, the need for story-lines to develop, peak and pass quite quickly may present a very unrealistic portrayal of an illness, how it develops over time and how it can affect someone's life.

Stigma

Stigma refers to an attribute that 'discredits', or prevents, someone's full acceptance in a particular situation.

Goffman is probably one of the best-known sociologists to have studied and theorised how certain groups of people attract stigma. His humanistic and sympathetic work focuses on why certain attributes of an individual or group deny them full acceptance in given situations and lead them either to be excluded or to be left with a feeling of not 'fitting in'. He classifies stigma into three broad groups:

- **physical stigma** – mainly to do with aspects visible 'on the surface' of people, for example facial scarring, a physical impairment or an amputation
- **personal/character stigma** – mainly to do with aspects 'below the surface', for example drug use, sexuality or mental health
- **social stigma** – belonging to a particular group or ethnic minority. (Goffman, 1968)

Question

Can you identify conditions, mental or physical, that could be potentially stigmatising? Try to figure out why they could be stigmatising?

Like other symbolic interactionists, Goffman seeks to explore the subtleties and intricacies of how people present themselves to the outside world, especially if their identity is in some way 'spoiled' or stigmatised. How that identity can be spoiled or stigmatised varies greatly. Sometimes it is highly visible, in the case of facial scarring for example, or it can be highly invisible, such as a history of depressive episodes. Whatever it is, it may completely alter social identity. In some respects we all have something in our lives that we wish to keep hidden, or pieces of personal information that we manage in certain ways so as to maintain a particular 'face' to those about us.

Another aspect of Goffman's notion of stigma is that it is highly relational, depending on the situation in which we find ourselves. The previous section outlined how people experiencing mental health problems are portrayed in a negative light, and, if their status is known, in certain situations the effects could be quite damaging. If, let us say, that person was, for example, with others who shared similar mental health problems then the stigma would be reduced or non-existent. Notions of what is normal, or what stigma is, are thus highly contextual with each of these labels being socially constructed with no inherent or natural basis.

People respond in a variety of ways to a potentially stigmatising condition or situation though, as Goffman argues, this can depend on how concealed or 'displayed' the stigma is. For those with a concealed or concealable stigma, an attribute that Goffman terms 'a discreditable stigma', there is the possibility of managing, manipulating or presenting information so as to avoid revealing the stigma. This is termed **passing** and entails devising a routine. This routine may involve being careful about what one talks about, where one goes, what one wears and so on – basically managing daily life so as to keep potentially stigmatising information secret.

Goffman points out that trying to maintain this round of secrecy can come at a terrible cost and be quite emotionally draining and demanding. There is always the chance of letting information slip or being discovered, and the consequences, real or imagined, would then have to be endured.

As persuasive and elaborate as Goffman's ideas are, he has been criticised for not acknowledging the material basis of stigmas and for overly reflecting on the individual. His ideas do, however, provide a challenge to health professionals as he stresses the importance of constructing identity. As the work by Baker and MacPherson (2000) illustrates, the social stigma of a condition can at times be more of an issue for someone with a mental illness than the condition itself. We need to be aware of how the social framing of mental health and illness affects the lives of people who are experiencing distress.

Passing refers to attempts to conceal a potential stigma and prevent its disclosure.

Example of stigma and passing

Mary encountered severe mental health problems shortly after leaving university with a degree in plant science. Feeling very depressed, she found herself unable to leave her flat and even to attend to her personal hygiene. After several years of drug therapy and counselling she became more socially confident and able to deal with aspects of her mental health. She soon reached the point where she wanted to start working and perhaps catch up with old friends again. However, she did not want them to find out about her mental health problems and was worried that they might find her strange or dangerous. The potential problem was made worse by having a gap of several years in her life when she was ill and did not start a career like so many of her old university friends. Fortunately, she managed to find a job working in the greenhouses of the local botanical gardens. Her job involved routine repair and cleaning activities, even though she was qualified to take on more complex and demanding work. The job, though, gave Mary the cover of saying that she was working in the botanical gardens, making it sound as if she was currently in work of an appropriate level for a graduate with several years' work experience, even though it was not. This made it easier for her to catch up with old friends as she could pass herself as 'normal' and hide aspects of her biography that she did not want revealed.

9.3 Patterns of mental health/illness

As mentioned in the introduction, mental illness affects a wide cross-section of people of different ages, sexes and ethnicity. Nevertheless, certain conditions tend to be found in some groups more than in others and certain people, for a variety of reasons, are more at risk. Overall, mental illnesses are fairly common. The most widespread form of mental illness is depression. A summary of the statistics would indicate that:

- Around 300 people out of 1,000 will experience mental health problems every year in Britain
- 230 of these will visit a GP
- 102 will be diagnosed as having a mental health problem
- 24 will be referred to a specialist psychiatric service
- 6 will become in-patients in psychiatric services. (MIND 2000a)

It is quite apparent from Figure 9.1 and 9.2 that there is a tendency for mental illness to be distributed unevenly across the class scale, and in particular amongst women. In the research this association between social class and mental illness has long been noticeable. Early researchers such as Faris and Dunham (1939), in their study of the various residential zones of Chicago, observed that schizophrenia was more frequent among working-class people. Slightly later American work by Hollingshead and Redlich (1953) also identified class factors in relation to mental disorder. The now classic work by Brown and Harris (1978) similarly noted class differences: they came across higher rates of depression among working-class women with children than among their middle-class counterparts.

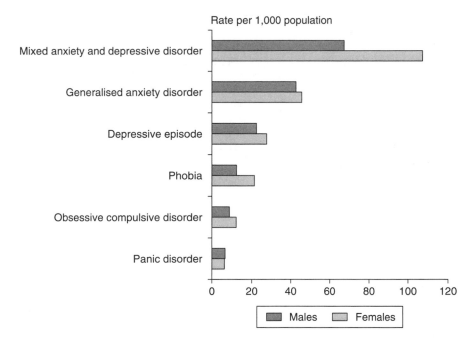

FIGURE 9.1   *Weekly prevalence of neurotic disorders: by sex, 2000. Great Britain (ONS 2006a)*
Source: National Statistics website: www.statistics.gov.uk
Crown copyright material is reproduced with the permission of the Controller of HMSO
Reproduced under the terms of the Click-Use Licence

9.4 Ethnicity and mental health

There are a number of explanations for why people from Black and other ethnic backgrounds appear to have higher rates of mental illness and a different, often coercive, relationship with services. These explanations include:

- racist and prejudiced attitudes on the part of service providers and agencies of the state, such as the police;
- lack of cultural sensitivity;
- more frequent exposure to stressors in the form of, for example, unemployment;
- adjusting to a new society if recently arrived;
- racism generally.

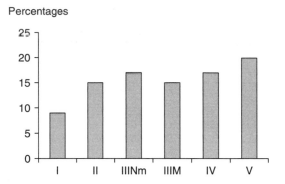

Percentages

FIGURE 9.2   *Prevalence of neurotic disorders: by social class, 2000. Great Britain (ONS 2004)*
Source: National Statistics website: www.statistics.gov.uk
Crown copyright material is reproduced with the permission of the Controller of HMSO
Reproduced under the terms of the Click-Use Licence

Links

These issues are discussed in greater depth in Chapter 7 on ethnicity and health.

These explanations are useful when trying to understand the situation of people from ethnic minorities in relation to mental illness. However, Pilgrim and Rogers (1993) point to another, related concept that may help us in this context. They draw on Foucault's concept of seeing madness as part of the 'other', that is, groups of people who are regarded as being outside the norms of society and as constituting a threat to the order of society. In previous times people with mental illnesses were excluded from society, banished to the Ships of Fools that traversed European waterways in the Middle Ages, or to the asylums of the Victorian age. Here we see, they argue, a relationship between new **racism** and psychiatric discourse. In the new racism many of the explicit old racist practices of viewing Black and Asian people as sub-human have given way to viewing people as a threat to 'British' social and cultural identity. This idea was noticeable during a speech made by Conservative MP John Townsend in the 2001 UK general election when he claimed that immigration was undermining Britain as an Anglo-Saxon country. The new racism also deals with this supposed threat to social and cultural identity by using exclusion, this time by excluding Black and Asian people from full social acceptance into British society on grounds of non-Christian religions, of diets, involvement in terrorism, or other 'non-western/British' aspects of identity behaviour. Thus, psychiatric practice reflects, in its treatment of Black and Asian wider aspects of racism within society by further excluding these groups from full social participation by identifying behaviour and activities as pathological and insane.

Gender refers to the cultural differences between men and women, while **sex** refers to physical differences.

9.5 Gender and mental health

Every review of the literature concerning sociology and mental health reaches the same conclusion when discussing gender – that women always display higher rates of certain mental illnesses than men (Foster 1995; Bebbington 1996). Much research has attempted to explain this particular phenomenon, with various results. Some explanations point to measurement artefact effects and to men seeking alternative outlets, such as drink, that mask depressive disorders; others point to role strain/conflict; while yet others indicate that social factors, such as poor housing or social class, are the cause. Other explanations point to the pressure on women to conform to prevailing norms of femininity and attractiveness. For example, the BMA (2000) warned that media images of very thin models and celebrities could have very damaging and negative effects on young women's perceptions of their body image and their self-esteem; which could lead to feelings of distress and anxiety.

Links

See Chapter 8 for more information on gender and health.

Measurement artefact means that women exhibit higher rates of mental illness than men because the design of questionnaires and the way in which data is collected produces a 'statistical mirage', which artificially generates a problem where there is not one. Earlier work by Gove (1984), among others, indicated that faults with the way in which data was collected meant that women appeared to exhibit higher rates of depression.

In a substantial review of the literature relating to women and depression, however, Bebbington (1996) and Nazroo et al. (1998) argued that there was little evidence of measurement artefact being responsible for the high levels of recorded depression in women. In their carefully constructed study, Nazroo et al. (1998) demonstrated that women did

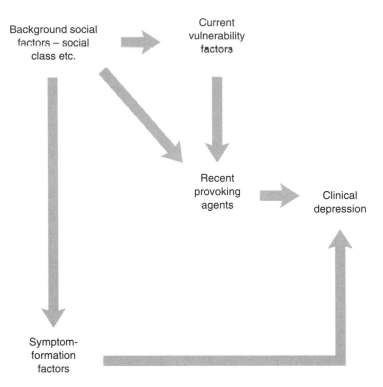

FIGURE 9.3   *Schematic representation of Brown and Harris' model of depression*
Source: Brown and Harris 1978: 265

report more depressive episodes – whether distant, mild or exaggerated episodes. There was little evidence for men masking their depression by turning to alcohol or substance abuse, as had been suggested by other studies.

What Nazroo et al.'s research pointed to was the effect that gender roles and life events had on men and women. Looking at a range of crises that related to children, reproduction, housing, finance, work, marital issues, crime and health, the researchers concluded that women were more likely to develop depression if a crisis involved children, housing or reproduction. The chance of depression was increased if a woman's role identity meant that she attached greater importance to those areas. So, if, for example, a women feels a particularly close attachment to and sense of responsibility for children because of her role identity, then the chance of depression is much greater if there is a child-related problem, such as difficulties at school or drug misuse. For crises involving finance or work, marital issues, crime or health, there appeared to be no gender role difference.

One of the best-known pieces of sociological research on women and mental health was carried out by Brown and Harris (1978), who sought to analyse the relationship between social factors and mental health in the Camberwell area of London. From their research they developed a multifactorial model, which attempted to explain the intricacies and subtleties of why some women develop clinical depression while others, living in similar conditions, do not. The model contains the idea that the onset of depression (the dependent variable) will occur if other factors are present (the independent variable). Key components of the model are:

- **current vulnerability factors** – these factors relate to events that have happened in a woman's past and indicate whether or not she may be more susceptible to depression. Brown and Harris identified four vulnerability factors:

  1 losing a mother before the age of 11;
  2 presence at home of three or more children under the age of 15 years;
  3 absence of any confiding relationships, particularly with the husband;
  4 lack of full- or part-time job.

- **provoking agents** – here Brown and Harris identified various events that could occur in a woman's life, which could then trigger a depressive episode. The events mainly relate to loss and disappointment, e.g. death, losing a job or discovering a partner's unfaithfulness. Ongoing difficulties were also noted as being contributory; they included dealing with a variety of 'background' problems ranging from housing difficulties to headaches.
- **symptom-formation factors** – women over 50 years of age and women with low self-esteem were at greatest risk of developing depression.

One way of thinking about this approach is to imagine someone on a tightrope. The chances of falling are increased if there are any existing vulnerabilities, which means that the tightrope begins to sway, making it harder to maintain a sure footing. There is an even greater chance of falling if a provoking agent such as an adverse life event comes along and impacts on the person, making it likely that they will be knocked off. Finally, any possibility of staying on the rope may be diminished if balance is poor due to low self-esteem.

9.6 Focus on depression

Depression is becoming an increasingly common condition in industrial capitalist societies, such as the UK. Psychologist Oliver James (1998) points to the increases in the amount of depression in British society since the 1950s. He goes on to make the highly apposite point that even though we are now, in many ways, richer economically we are definitely poorer emotionally. This, he argues, is due to the tendency of contemporary society (mainly through hyped-up media images) to heighten our expectations of what life should be about – expectations which are ultimately impossible to fulfil. This leads to a depressing 'gap' between where we think we should be in life and where we actually are, or, as James puts it, we think we are losers even though we are winners.

One problem, when discussing 'depression', is the term itself. In lay usage we use the word to describe and refer to a vast variety of states and feelings in everyday life. So, for example, you could claim to be feeling depressed after your football team loses yet again on a Saturday afternoon, or when the essay you feverishly worked on receives a lower grade than you'd hoped. The emotional states indicated in these two examples will be highly unpleasant, perhaps leading to some, albeit temporary, change in behaviour; for example, having a cry or wanting to be on your own. This is quite different from what is meant by experiencing depression as a mental illness. By confusing the states of everyday blues and the illness of depression many of the subtleties and issues which face people with clinical depression are lost. The severity of the condition and the experiences that people with depression go through may be unfairly diminished and not taken as seriously as they would be if the person was, for instance, experiencing a severe physical illness instead.

Depression is, therefore, considerably more than feeling just a little down or blue: people with clinical depression experience a highly distressing and debilitating combination of mental *and* physical symptoms that can last over a period of months or even years. In terms of mental states and emotions, people with depression have a substantial reordering of how they think, see themselves and perceive others. Thinking changes in that they interpret the world around very negatively and see everything in the worst possible and most despairing way. Frequently, people with depression are acutely sensitive to the smallest of things. So, for example, if a friend does not sit next to them in a lecture this can be taken as a sign that nobody likes them and that life is terrible. What is important here is that this change in thinking cannot be 'snapped out of', as is sometimes popularly thought. Such changes in thinking often seem beyond the control of the person with depression. They wish they could stop thinking in in such a negative and horrible way but find it almost impossible to do so. The following quote from someone with depression illustrates this point:

> It is so total … . There is no reason to wake up in the morning. I just let the blinds stay down … . Sometimes I wonder what life will be like, where I can find a fixed point, a hold to my life. (Kangas 2001: 86)

At worst, changes in thinking can take the direction of suicidal thoughts where taking one's life begins to appear as a 'suitable' way of dealing with life's problems. These thoughts are deeply despairing. We examine sociological perspectives on suicide in section 9.7. As well as all the changes in thinking there are also considerable physical changes. Among the more common changes that affect the body are exhaustion, difficulties in sleeping, loss of appetite, loss of weight, and loss of interest in **sex**. These physical changes indicate how the differences between physical and mental illness are not so clear-cut. Just because something is mainly seen as a mental illness does not mean that it is only experienced as a set of feelings. The same also goes for physical illnesses, which often have an emotional side to them too.

Throughout this chapter, there has been reference to how society views or frames mental illness. Depression is no exception and there are considerable cultural differences in how people from a particular society frame this mental illness. In an American study, Karasz (2005) found that there were differences between European Americans and South Asian immigrants in how they viewed depression. Two key differences emerged. The European Americans were more likely to see depression as a disease and a medical condition, not related to any social context, while the South Asians had the opposite viewpoint; they saw depression more as an emotional response to what was going on in someone's life and tied very closely to social context. Other social and cultural differences have been noted elsewhere. Fenton and Sadiq-Sangster (1996) found that South Asian women expressed depression in physical terminology, for example saying that they had a pain in their heart with little or no allusion to feelings or thoughts. What should be noted here is that just because different cultures frame depression in different ways does not mean that one is more accurate and correct than the other. All that this demonstrates is how social influences affect our ways of expressing our moments of suffering and anguish.

9.7 Suicide

On 8 April 1994 musician Kurt Cobain decided to take his own life and joined the list of various rock stars who have died early. His death was not an isolated tragedy, a one-off, but an instance of a trend that had been growing from the 1990s onwards: the increase in young male suicide. Even though suicide rates as a whole are down from the early 1980s, the suicide rate for young men has increased since 1982 by 67 per cent for young men aged 15–24, accounting for 20 per cent of all deaths for young people in that age group (MIND 1999). The highest rate for suicide though, is still found among older men (ibid.). Suicide often appears to be an unfathomable act, impervious to **analysis** or systematic understanding. After all, how can any research be carried out on an action that takes place in isolated and lonely circumstances, where the subject is someone whose life has reached the place where ending it appears a valid choice?

Question

Do you think that there is glamour attached to the suicides of successful artistic people? If so why?

Links

Chapter 1, section 1.2 discusses functionalism in more depth.

There has been much (perhaps too much, some would say) sociological work on suicide, mainly because of early work by functionalist Emile Durkheim. Durkheim used suicide as an example of how the most apparently individual of acts can be opened up to sociological investigation. First published in 1897, *Suicide: A Study in Sociology*, was the first sociological attempt to systematically understand suicide (Durkheim 1970). Without denying that individual circumstances could affect a person's decision to take his or her own life, Durkheim noticed patterns in suicide rates between countries and between different groups in the same society. Protestant countries had higher rates than Catholic countries, while Jewish societies had the lowest suicide rates of all. What was also notable was the constancy of relative suicide rates between countries. After further analysis Durkheim identified four different types of suicide:

- **Egoistic suicide**: If an individual was not sufficiently integrated into society then they were at a higher risk of suicide. This explains why Protestants were at greater risk than Catholics. The Protestant faith emphasises individualism, while Catholicism emphasises community, with greater integration for a community's members. In addition, people who were unmarried or childless were more likely to commit suicide than the married and those with children, because of the former's lack of integration with a family unit.
- **Anomic suicide**: The opposite of egoistic suicide, this occurs where a society fails to regulate the individual, for example when a society collapses and all the usual norms and patterns of life fall apart, leaving people bewildered and unsure of what is happening. The classic example of this is the 1928 stock market crash that just about devastated American life, with people losing security, savings and their homes. Here the loss of all that was considered normal led to an increase in suicide rates.

- **Altruistic suicide**: Here a sense of duty, linked to a high level of integration into a particular society, leads someone to take their own life. There are numerous examples around the world: the Japanese kamikaze pilots who flew their planes directly into American battleships in an attempt to sink them during the Second World War; the Hindu practice of suttee, where a wife kills herself at her husband's funeral; and the Irish Republican hunger strikers, such as Bobby Sands, who starved themselves to death in pursuit of their political beliefs.
- **Fatalistic suicide**: This form of suicide refers to the despair of living in a highly regulated society with no opportunity for personal freedom and control. It is very rare in contemporary society and Durkheim only included it for historical interest. Mainly applying to highly restrictive societies, this type of suicide could be seen among slaves in ancient slave societies.

As with any other groundbreaking and important piece of sociology Durkheim's theory of suicide has attracted much debate, with many proponents and opponents. Some critics point out that suicide statistics are notoriously unreliable. Coroners or doctors may record a death as due to some cause other than suicide, in an attempt to avoid problems for surviving family members. Other critics pointed out that his observations could not always be proved or researched properly.

The strongest critique, however, came from interpretative sociologists such as J.D. Douglas (1967). He put forward two points:

1   All suicide statistics should be treated with caution, as there may have been collusion between officials who record and categorise deaths, and family and friends. The degree of integration here may affect the decision. The more integrated the suicide in a social group, the greater the possibility of a cover-up taking place.
2   Durkheim failed to take into account the motive for and meaning of the suicide. Suicide can be a way of communicating revenge, eliciting sympathy or dealing with guilt, or a way of meeting cultural obligations. This information could be elicited by studying diaries and suicide notes.

Links

Chapter 1, section 1.2 discusses interpretative perspectives in greater depth.

More recent sociologists have criticised theories of the interpretative approach of sociologists such as Douglas, and sought to construct more elegant and sophisticated theories of suicide. Taylor (1989, 1990) also agreed that statistics are unreliable and noted, in a study of deaths in the London Underground, a number of contributory factors that could lead to a death being recorded as a suicide, or not. These included whether or not the person had a history of mental illness, or the views and opinions of people who knew the deceased. If the coroner asked a close friend or family member then suicide would often be denied, while if the coroner asked a casual acquaintance, a verdict of suicide was be more likely.

Taylor then went on to identify four different types of suicide. This categorisation is similar to Durkheim's, but Taylor's emphasis is less on social factors and more on what people think of themselves and their relationships with others, and how certain or uncertain these feelings are is what is important here. These suicides divide into two main categories: ectopic, which relates to a person's view of him/herself; and symphisic, that is concerning the person's relationship with others.

Ectopic suicides (self)

Submissive suicide – occurs when someone has decided that there is no point in going on and that their life is at an end. This may be because of the death of a loved one, or because of terminal illness. Any attempt at suicide is carried out with the full intention of taking one's life and may take place in an isolated place so as to avoid the chance of discovery.

Thanatation suicide – relates to feelings of uncertainty, and the attempt at suicide is not as earnest as a submissive suicide, the person leaving it to chance as to whether they actually die or not.

Symphisic suicide (relationships)

Sacrifice suicides – here the person takes their own life in order to make others, such as partners or former lovers, feel guilty or incur censure from friends and family. Any suicide note will indicate on whom the blame for the suicide rests.

Appeal suicide – this occurs when someone is uncertain how others feel about them. The person who attempts suicide is not necessarily trying to end their life, but testing the reactions of others. The suicide attempt may be staged in such a way, in front of others for example, as to enable the person who is making the attempt to see how much someone else cares about them.

Questions

Which of the above theories do you find the most satisfactory in attempting to explain suicide? Provide justification for your answer.

The above three sociological theories of suicide present interesting and different perspectives on why people decide to take their own lives. Each has a particular strength or weakness, and in many ways a combination of all three provides some useful insights into why people attempt suicide. Durkheim offers useful ideas on how social pressures and wider aspects of a society affect suicidal behaviour, while Douglas cautions against accepting suicide statistics at face value and urges us to look at meaning. In Taylor's work we find explanations of why some people leave notes, or attempt suicide in a variety of locations with different levels of secrecy or openness.

Conclusion

A theme running through this chapter has been how distress, suffering and mental health issues are framed and very much influenced by society. This extends from trying to define what is meant by mental illness and the ways in which wider attitudes (and prejudices) impinge on official discourses and perspectives, to the difficult experiences of people with mental health problems and the ways in which they can be stigmatised by wider society. Indeed, for many people who feel depressed or experience other issues with their mental and emotional well-being it is the reactions of others that can cause them more problems in their day-to-day lives.

We have seen once more that, as with other aspects of health, there exist great social inequalities. Women, working-class people and people from minority ethnic groups all appear to report higher levels of distress. Again, social influences are at play here. We can see the pressures created by expectations of what it is to be feminine, the experience of stress and poverty, or the consequences of racism all having potential negative consequences. This chapter has highlighted that mental health has to be understood in its widest context, with sociology providing insights into the social processes that influence and define the misery and suffering of many people in society today.

Given the higher profile of mental health issues and well-being in contemporary society it appears that interventions in improving and maintain good mental health have to take place at a social level just as much, if not more, than at a personal level.

SUMMARY POINTS

- Mental illness, particularly depression, is common in contemporary society.
- Many people hold negative images of mental illness. These negative images often associate mental illness with danger, whether to others or to the mentally ill person. Media portrayals of mental illness are often similarly negative. The stigma created by negative images can have an adverse impact on people with mental illness.
- Ethnic minorities have a different experience of mental health care than do White people. African-Caribbean young men are more likely to be perceived as difficult or violent and more likely to enter mental health care via the police. Cultural stereotyping and racist attitudes affect the care of people from ethnic backgrounds. This also includes white ethnic groups, such as Irish people.
- Women have a different experience of mental health care and mental illness from men. Women tend to have higher rates of depression than men. Stress created by attachment to gender roles is likely to be the cause of those higher rates.
- Overall suicide rates are decreasing but suicide rates for young men aged 15–24 are increasing. Various sociological theories point to a variety of reasons as to why people take their own lives. Durkheim stresses social and cultural factors. Douglas warns against accepting statistics at face value and emphasises the need to understand individual meaning, while Taylor looks at feelings of uncertainty and certainty with self and others.

Case study

John has recently been relocated into a community hostel that helps those with a variety of mild and non-violent mental illnesses to reintegrate into society. The hostel is situated in a reasonably affluent suburb near a sizeable public park.

It was during his fourth year at university that John first came into contact with the psychiatric services. Up till then John was a fairly standard student, competent but not especially noteworthy. This was probably due to his participation in a rather hectic social life of which he appeared to be one of the prime movers. This particular group of friends clubbed quite extensively at the weekends and some of the group took drugs. As he himself remarked to a case worker: 'Yeah, drugs were part of what we did at the weekends but it was nothing serious – dope mainly and speed. Well, speed most Fridays and Saturdays just to help us get that extra energy boost.'

In his third year one of this group was killed in a random accident. They had been out on a Friday night and John had encouraged everyone to try and drink and smoke as much dope as possible. After the club had closed they headed down to the nearby beach to watch the sun come up. It was there that John's friend slipped on a rock and fell to his death. Strong feelings of guilt overcame John as he felt to blame for the accident. He gradually became more withdrawn from his friends, and his use of alcohol and soft drugs increased. At the start of his fourth year a relationship with another student fell apart. She found his increasingly pessimistic moods difficult to handle. In addition, his overall behaviour was becoming more compulsive – he constantly analysed what lay behind her words and actions. Invariably, all his conclusions were negative and he firmly believed that she was bored with him. After she left he ceased attending classes and his coursework suffered. He spent most of his time in his flat, unable to sleep and constantly fixating on what he had done wrong in his life. One night in an attempt to sleep he drank half a bottle of whisky and took some sleeping tablets. A flatmate found him unconscious on the living-room floor and rushed him to hospital.

In the following weeks he was advised to see a counsellor and was refered to cognitive therapy. He made some progress, but as the year went on his university friends finished their courses and moved out of the area. This left John feeling alone and isolated.

Consequently his problems returned, and this time he was placed in the local psychiatric hospital. The seven months that he spent there seem to have made some difference to him. In his stay there he responded well to medication and to the various therapies, and hints of his former self appeared. At various social events the charismatic aspects of his personality, which had been quite strong during his university days, surfaced. However, the outside world still seemed problematic to him and he found it difficult to be among large groups of people on his own. In addition to this he had nowhere to stay, as he was no longer entitled to student accommodation.

It was then decided that the hostel was the best place for him as his family might find it difficult to care for him. His father had left home to set up a new life for himself and his new partner, a former office colleague, and his parents divorced. As a result of the separation John's mother developed a severe long-term depression and found life generally difficult to cope with. Recently she had been experiencing some ill-effects from a course of Fluoxetine prescribed by her doctor. This led to her taking several days off work from the department store she worked in. Management were reasonably supportive but proposed restructuring of the department was causing her some anxiety because of the possible loss of a part-time assistant, which would increase her workload. It was proposed that his father might help to care for him, but John did not feel that he was ready to re-establish such a relationship with his father as he still felt some ambivalence towards him for leaving the family home.

Life at the hostel had until recently been going reasonably well. John was managing to socialise again and felt confident about interacting with the world at large. In fact, he had managed to get to know some local people his own age. They knew he was at the hostel but he claimed that he was a worker there and with his quick wit and outward appearance of calm there was no reason to doubt this. However, one day in the nearby supermarket John suddenly felt quite anxious and rushed out of the store, discarding his shopping as he left. This was witnessed by one of his new friends who started to have doubts about John's true identity.

1   Discuss how John's sense of identity has been affected by his mental illness. How important is maintaining a sense of identity for John?
2   What has happened in his mother's life that has led her to feel depressed? Which theory could help us understand her situation?
3   What passing technique does John employ?
4   If you are a health professional student what type of involvement would you have with someone like John?
5   The assumption is that John is White, but how might his treatment and subsequent care and recovery have been different if he was a young African-Caribbean male?

Taking your studies further

This chapter will have helped you understand many of the key terms, concepts, theories and debates relating to mental health. Listed below are journal articles and books that will provide deeper and more detailed discussions of the points raised in this chapter. You will also find what is available on the companion website. This offers you downloads of relevant material, plus links to useful websites in addition to podcasts and other features.

Recommended reading

Books

Busfield, J. (ed.) (2001) *Rethinking the Sociology of Mental Health* (Sociology of Health and Illness Monographs). London: Blackwell.

Goffman, E. (1968) *Stigma: Notes on the Management of a Spoiled Identity.* Harmondsworth: Penguin.

Philo, G. (ed.) (1996) *Media and Mental Distress.* London: Longman.

Pilgrim, D. (2005) *Key Concepts in Mental Health.* London: Sage.

Pilgrim, D. and Rogers, A. (2005) *A Sociology of Mental Health and Illness.* Buckingham: Open University Press.

Prior, L. (1993) *The Social Organization of Mental Illness.* London: Sage.

Journal article

Pilgrim, D. and Bentall, R. (1999) 'The medicalisation of misery: a critical realist analysis of the concept of depression', *Journal of Mental Health,* 8 (3): 261–74.

Website

The MIND website has a wealth of useful and interesting information: http://www.mind.org.uk/

On the companion website

Muntaner, C., Eaton, W.W. and Diala, C.C. (2000) 'Social inequalities in mental health: a review of concepts and underlying assumptions', *Health,* 4 (1): 89–113.

10

Sociology of the body: chronic illness and disability

MAIN POINTS

- The body is not simply a biological entity only understood by the natural sciences.
- Perceptions of the body, what we do with our bodies and how the body is regulated are all influenced by society.
- Morality is attached to the presentation of the body in contemporary society, with thin bodies perceived as being 'good' and overweight bodies perceived as 'bad'.
- Chronic illness leads to 'biographical disruption', where the 'taken-for-granted' aspects of life and identity are thrown into question.
- The medical model of disability locates the causes of disability in the individual body.
- The social model of disability sees the causes of disability as a form of social oppression and discrimination.

KEY CONCEPTS

The sociology of the body, embodiment, the civilised body, identity, chronic illness, normality, stigma, biographical disruption.

Introduction

The sociology of the body addresses how we use our bodies, how we engage with them and, fundamentally, seeks to understand the nature of the physical body. The key point to bear in mind is that the body is both 'natural' and the product of its social environment.

This chapter concentrates on the *sociology of the body* and what it can contribute to our understanding of health and illness. While there will be a strong emphasis on a theoretical approach to the human body, there will be equal coverage of the significance of **embodiment** through an examination of the impact of living with chronic illness and disability.

10.1 Key issues in the study of the body

Until relatively recently sociologists shied away from theorising and researching the human body. This reluctance is twofold. First, there is an unwillingness to be caught up in biological and determinist explanations of human behaviour. Sociologists have, for example, chosen to study **gender** rather than **sex** differences, since the latter is often used to defend inequalities between women and men. The concept of gender, on the other hand, removes the problem of the bodily differences and draws our attention to the social construction of the terms 'male' and 'female' in terms of the values, beliefs and expectations placed on biological women and men. The second explanation for the general reluctance to embrace the body stems from the historical and cultural origins of the discipline itself. As the opening chapter illustrated, the founding fathers of **sociology** were primarily concerned to explain the social changes brought about by urbanisation and industrialisation. Early sociological texts indicate a preoccupation with topics such as urbanisation, religion, paid work and the role of the state. Physical differences between people mattered less than inequalities of **class** and status. Differences such as those between women and men and between adults and children were seen as belonging to the 'natural' world, and were unchangeable and fixed. In recent times, however, sociology has developed to include topics such as sex and gender, disability, and the physical and biological aspects of our lives. In addition to changes within the discipline of sociology, a number of social and cultural shifts have taken place which have resulted in a renewed interest in the human body. The body has ceased to be the preserve of the medical and scientific world and has become a major concern for sociologists. Figure 10.1 illustrates the main trends and developments.

Bodies are central to everything that we do and yet this centrality seems to have resulted in attitudes that very much take the body for granted; the body is so obvious it is hardly worth comment.

Body politics: Recognition that the physical body has a social and political status such that a different body (whether that is female as opposed to male, or a body with a disability) helps determine an individual's life chances. The feminist movement and the disability movement have played a central role in attempting to ensure that people have power over their own bodies.

Demographic changes: An increasingly ageing population draws attention to the physical changes arising from the ageing process and the consequences of living with an ageing body.

The prevalence of chronic illnesses: There has been a significant change in what Nettleton and Watson refer to as 'the disease burden'. Infectious diseases have now been replaced by chronic and degenerative conditions, many of which raise important questions about how a physically changed body impacts on our sense of identity and how people live with pain and discomfort.

Consumerism: An increased emphasis on the appearance and health of the body- People are concerned about maintaining their bodies in good condition and purchasing goods to help them do so. In this context, 'good' suggests youthful, slim and active.

Technological changes: Physical limitations of the body can be overcome, appearance can be changed, organs and limbs repaired and replaced. It becomes increasingly difficult to distinguish between the 'natural' body and the 'technological' body.

The body as an expression of our identity: The body becomes a means to express an identity. Diet, exercise and lifestyles can be portrayed as 'moral' or 'immoral' and 'irresponsible'.

FIGURE 10.1   *Bringing the body to the fore*
Source: adapted from Nettleton and Watson (1998: 4)

If one thing is certain, it is that we all have a body. Everything that we do we do with our bodies — when we think, speak, listen, eat, sleep, walk, relax, work and play we 'use' our bodies. Every aspect of our lives is therefore embodied. Sometimes we may be more aware of our bodies than others but from the moment we wake, we are to a greater or lesser extent, consciously or sub-consciously relying on our bodies. (Nettleton and Watson 1998: 1)

Because of the fundamentality of the body it is of undoubted interest for students of sociology generally, and students of the sociology of health in particular. For Shilling, the human body marks the boundary between ourselves and others; it is a means of presenting 'both the uniqueness of each individual and a site for the marking of difference' (Shilling 1997: 65). Some of the most obvious differences to consider are those of gender, **race** and levels of physical ability, but the body may also be adorned with certain clothes (or not), paints, tattoos or ornaments. Shilling also observes that, over and above our own interest in our bodies, many professional groups in contemporary **society** are also concerned with the body. Clinicians, psychologists, social workers and physical educationalists take the body and what happens to it as their legitimate concern and intervene in the way in which we see our own bodies (ibid.). Ultimately the body is *the* subject of all research and work relating to medicine and health (Lupton 1995). Understanding, shaping and intervening in the body are all central themes of this book – for example, in relation to the discussion of women's reproductive capacity. Control over the techniques of reproduction makes possible control over bodies, what happens to them, when, and how.

We have highlighted the significance of the body as a subject for students of sociology by emphasising the central role played by our physical selves in all that we do. Sociologists also seek to 'see' the body in more than purely physical and biological terms, drawing our attention to the two key 'social' aspects of the body. The first of these is the impact of environmental, cultural, social and political influences on the body, while the second aspect is the knowledge that the body is shaped by certain dominant discourses such as medicine. Chapter 6 examines inequalities in health and presents evidence that indicates a relationship between social class and patterns of morbidity and mortality. Social class can be used as an indicator of the types of illnesses people experience, as well as their life expectancy. Historical evidence reveals that body shape and stature are influenced by environmental factors. Birke (1992: 74–5) suggests an almost circular process where biology (A), environment (B) and the outcome (C) all interact to transform one another. In her example, genetic inheritance interacts with nutrition to produce the final height of a child. Importantly, however, the final height of the child then influences the genes he or she passes on, which then interact with the environment – and so the process goes on. The second sense in which sociologists understand the body is in terms of our knowledge of the social construction of the physical. There is an inherent danger in understanding the body as only a social construction as this may impede the study of the body as a real and physical entity. Nettleton and Watson (1998: 2) point to a tendency for the sociology of the body to suffer from theoreticism, where there is little or no reference to the empirical evidence about the lived experience of *embodiment*. This chapter will overcome this with a detailed consideration of the embodied experience of living with chronic illness.

> **Question**
>
> *Can you identify how and when you are most aware of your body.*

10.2 The civilised body: a controlled body and a 'clean' body

This section seeks to explore concepts of privacy and of the civilised, clean body. Views on what is appropriate bodily behaviour and who has access to our bodies

Embodiment refers to the experience of living through and with the physical body. Our experiences are essentially embodied. For example we experience pleasure and pain through the body. Feelings of happiness and sadness are as physical as they are emotional

The concept of the **civilised body** was developed by Norbert Elias. The term is used to denote a historical and cultural shift whereby the body is subject to increasing restraints that appear to limit the 'natural' body. The development of rules around eating manners is an example of how the body has become 'civilised'.

have a key bearing on the delivery of health care as well as on our experience of illness. The physical examination of the body is central to the practice of medicine: it is this that allows practitioners to investigate whether or not the body is functioning normally. Doctors, nurses, physiotherapists, opticians and dentists are all required to touch the body, sometimes in intimate ways. Illness often entails losing some control over bodily functions. Migraine, for example, can cause uncontrollable vomiting, and food poisoning can lead to uncontrollable diarrhoea. Physical incapacity can necessitate the use of a commode, thus requiring someone to share what is not only an intimate act but also one that has overtones of being unclean. How we negotiate access to other bodies and how we think of our own are, therefore, key issues for the sociology of health.

As Nettleton and Watson (1998) have stated, we all have bodies and everything that we do we do through them. All bodies have the same basic needs in terms of food, water and sleep. We must all remove waste from our bodies in the form of urine and faeces. Whether through illness or over-indulgence, our bodies vomit and we have little control over this. All bodies have the same basic components but differ in size, shape and colour. These are all fundamental human experiences and activities and yet, particularly in contemporary western societies, the body and its functions are regarded with a degree of shame and embarrassment.

To explore these concepts in more depth we will examine the work of Norbert Elias, first published in 1939, in relation to manners and the development of 'civilised' society. Elias' (1982) historical account of the **civilised body** examines the development of preferred ways of behaving and of control over the physical functions of the body. Regulation of the body came to be associated with higher social status and refinement. Nettleton (1995: 116–17) argues that the civilising of the body involves three progressive elements:

Socialisation:	People learn to conceal the natural functions of the body. We come to 'know' that certain functions such as defecating or vomiting are essentially private and potentially distasteful to others.
Rationalisation:	We prize our ability to control our emotions. Anger may be felt but only expressed in an acceptable way.
Individualisation:	Individual bodies are seen as separate from others. We demand a degree of personal 'social space' and privacy.

The development of ideas about the civilised body also demonstrates a concern to distinguish between human and bestial behaviour (Hawkes 1996: 20) and accords with Enlightenment notions about the higher self being associated with the mind, and the base self with the body.

The work of Elias helps us to understand why people find intimate medical examination potentially embarrassing and why an inability to control the basic functions of the body can lead to stigmatisation. Control over our most basic bodily functions is something we require even in young children. As Nettleton suggests above, **socialisation** into the norms of any society entails learning that certain types of behaviour are private and potentially shameful when performed inappropriately. Mayall (1996) notes that much of the socialisation process is about teaching children to control their bodies and to be civilised. Young children are taught appropriate table manners, toilet trained, and taught the necessity of sitting still in preparation for schooling. Even at an early age, then, the importance of bodily control is underlined. Equally, the essentially private nature of the naked body and of sex is an implicit part of the concept of the civilised body. In her study of sex and sexuality, Hawkes argues that in medieval times nudity was not a source of shame and that sexual matters were discussed without any sense of embarrassment. She notes, too, that accompanying 'couples to the marital bed and celebration of the consummation were customs that persisted well into the seventeenth century' (Hawkes 1996: 22). After that period both nudity and sexual matters were moved 'behind the scenes', appropriate only in private (ibid.: 23).

Question

Identify examples of when the body is subject to regulation and control, in both medical and non-medical settings.

How then do health practitioners deal with the potential discomfort that arises from physically intimate examinations? According to Lawler (1991), nursing staff have adopted a number of strategies to cope with potential embarrassment and shame, both on their part and on the part of the patient. There are a number of rules that appear to govern such encounters. The first is that patients should comply with requests for examinations because they are dependent on nursing staff. Here it is helpful to refer back to Parsons' model of **the sick role** because it too justifies access to the patient's body on the grounds of expertise on the part of the practitioner. In addition, the practitioner's own professional code of conduct is, arguably, meant to protect the patient from potential abuse and exploitation. By maintaining a degree of professional distance, the situation may be depersonalised. Lawler (1991) also argues that patients themselves are expected to maintain a degree of modesty, while the nurse attempts to protect the patient's privacy.

Maintaining personal hygiene when ill often requires assistance with bathing but it is common for nursing staff to allow patients the option of cleaning their own private parts. It is ironic that while much of modern health care is premised on practices such as holistic care, being attended to by a named carer, and attempts generally to break down the barriers between patients and staff, it seems that there are some circumstances when a professional and distanced stance is appreciated by both parties.

Question

What are your experiences either as a patient being examined or as a practitioner undertaking an examination of a patient?

Chapter 3 dealt with the subject of the new public health movement, emphasising the extent to which governments are concerned with controlling individual bodies as well as the social body. Behind these developments lies the fear that without regulation bodies would be out of control. Disease and contamination of the body have been central concerns of the public health movement. Lupton (1995), for example, writes of the economic and political implications of disease in terms of absence from work.

Our discussion of **medicalisation** illustrated the way in which it is not just unhealthy bodies that come under the scrutiny of the medical profession; there is an important sense in which we are all judged to be 'at risk'. The issues of cleanliness and hygiene are important illustrations of this trend, because there is considerable emphasis on preserving health through cleanliness. Lupton (1995) provides an interesting historical account of just how our concept of cleanliness has changed over time:

> Consider the following examples of how, at varying periods in time, the body was kept clean and safe from infection and make a note of your personal reactions to them: Being 'clean' meant that those areas of the body seen by others were free of dirt. Washing was 'dry' in the sense that a cloth was used to rub the face and hands.
>
> Bathing was not an option; immersing the body in water was thought to weaken it as the liquid might invade the body.
>
> Once bathing became an accepted practice cold bathing was preferred as it was thought to toughen and invigorate the body.
>
> The use of 'cosmetics' such as perfume to scent the body was seen as frivolous. (Lupton 1995: 33–4)

These examples of hygienic practices are in marked contrast to the values prevalent in most western societies. Personal hygiene is both desirable and, it might be argued, possible with the provision of indoor plumbing. We all sweat as a means of cooling the body down, yet the smell of sweat is shunned. Instead, we attempt either to prevent our bodies sweating (through the use of an anti-perspirant) or to mask the smell if the body does sweat (through the use of deodorant). Media images reinforce the message that bodies that are clean and perfumed are desirable bodies.

The desire for cleanliness extends beyond our bodies to our homes. The nineteenth-century push to improve the health of the nation focused primarily on instructing mothers in childcare practices and, significantly, in domestic hygiene. According to Hawkes (1996: 97) 'a good mother kept a clean home. Whiter whites were a sign of superiority.' The multitude of products that claim to be anti-bacterial or effective in combating the invisible threat of germs bears testimony to our fear of dirt and the negative moral connotations that attach to a lack of hygiene. Lupton argues that modern standards and beliefs about cleanliness are characterised by a fear of invisible germs and viruses. She comments in particular on a near obsession with the cleanliness of toilets and the desire to have a visible indication of cleanliness 'displayed by a bright blue chemical being released every time the lavatory is flushed' (Lupton 1995: 35).

Among commentators on the sociology of the body, it appears to be accepted that we as a population are obsessed with hygiene and cleanliness. There is some evidence to suggest that this view is simplistic. Recent outbreaks of salmonella and the spread of hospital-acquired infections have revealed hygiene practices that are far from perfect. Professor Hugh Pennington of the Bacteriology Department of Aberdeen University has been particularly critical of poor hygiene practices around the home. Among his main concerns is the use of washing-up bowls and re-usable dishcloths.

Professor Pennington said that placing chopping boards and knives teeming with germs together with plates and glasses in a plastic bowl created the ideal environment for the spread of bugs.

The experts said disposable paper cloths should be used instead of tea towels that could easily spread infection.

They also recommended using 'good old fashioned bleach' in the kitchen rather than newer anti-bacterial products that were only vaguely effective. (www.news.bbc.co.uk 2002)

The beginning of 2002 heralded a major health crisis for hospitals in Scotland as hospital-acquired infections in general and the MRSA bug in particular led to the closure of the Victoria Infirmary, Glasgow, to all new admissions. Once again, the problem appeared to be poor hygiene practices. Hugh Pennington commented that infection control was being severely compromised by lack of basic hygiene practices, such as doctors and nurses failing to wash their hands between treating patients.

The discussion above has highlighted the ways in which bodily functions and intimate access to the body can present barriers in the caring relationship. It has been suggested that shame and embarrassment about the body are not natural but are socially cultivated, and the work of Elias has provided an insight into the development of concepts of the 'civilised body'. Our discussion now takes us on to images and perceptions of the 'perfect' body.

10.3 The sculptured body: creating perfection

Images of bodily perfection, most often images of women, are powerful but never static. Whether it is the voluptuous bust, tiny waist and rounded bottom of the nineteenth century, the androgynous figure of the 1920s, the curves of Marilyn Monroe or the taut, lean and muscular body of Madonna, images of how female bodies should look are powerful reminders of the extent to which people have aspired to the perfect body. The purpose of this discussion is to examine how and why people have tried to attain that 'good' body. A later discussion of disability and chronic illness will pose powerful questions about what happens when bodies are not and cannot be made perfect.

Diet is perhaps the most obvious way in which we control the size and shape of the body. As Lupton comments: 'skin tone, weight, strength of bones, condition of hair and nails are all commonly said to be directly affected by diet' (Lupton 1995: 40). An increasingly important aspect of diet is the desire to limit the intake of food. Bordo argues that types of fasting have been common throughout history, and are usually characterised by control over the body's appetites or by a religious desire to purify the flesh (Bordo 1990: 83). However, she notes a significant shift during the late Victorian era, when, 'for the first time in the West, those who could afford to eat well began systematically to deny themselves food in the pursuit of an aesthetic ideal' (ibid.). So began what Bordo has described as the tyranny of slenderness.

In common with others, Bordo argues that body size is underpinned by a code of morality. The possession of a slender body suggests that the individual is in control of their body and their life. To achieve the 'perfect' body requires considerable time, effort and determination. Geri Halliwell recently achieved what she described as her ideal body; a body very much thinner than her previous form and made possible only with a strict diet and considerable time in the gym. In contrast, Helen Fielding's heroine, Bridget Jones, overeats, smokes and drinks in response to what she sees as an unfulfilled life. The actress who played Bridget Jones in the recent film soon shed the extra two stone put on for her role, reverting to her original size 6 in contrast to the 12 of the heroine. It is interesting to note that almost half of all women in Britain take a dress size 16 or over. Benson suggests that the body is increasingly seen as an indicator of a person's moral character.

The bad body is fat, slack, uncared for; it demonstrates a lazy and undisciplined 'self'. The good body is sleek, thin and toned. To have such a body is to project to those around you – as well as to yourself – that you are morally as well as physically 'in shape'. (Benson 1997: 123)

In the same vein, a muscular body has become what Bordo describes as a 'cultural icon':

The firm, developed body has become a symbol of correct *attitude;* it means that one 'cares' about oneself and how one appears to others, suggesting willpower, energy, control over infantile impulses, the ability to 'make something' of oneself. (Bordo 1990: 94–5)

Links

The desire (and ability) to control and discipline the body is seen as a characteristic of post-modern society. See Chapter 4.

Themes of controlling the body through will-power and discipline are frequent in accounts of people with eating disorders – a term which covers a range of behaviours from systematically starving the body, to overeating, and finally to eating and purging the body through vomiting or the use of laxatives. Although there is not the space here for a detailed discussion of eating disorders, a number of points can be made about the denial of food and the desire to assert power and autonomy. Benson (1997) describes the refusal to eat as 'an inescapably political act' because it is most often associated with asserting control and/or registering a protest. The use of hunger strikes as a political protest is common (Yuill 2007) and at the other end of the spectrum, a child's refusal to eat is a clear sign of defying parental authority. It has been suggested, therefore, that eating disorders such as anorexia may be a way of exercising power over the body, food intake being perhaps the only area of choice open to that person. Bordo examines limiting food intake in the context of a general cultural fear of 'fat' as an indicator of losing control over the body. In this sense, bodies have to be not only slender but contained, in the sense of minimising bulges and flab (Bordo 1990: 88–9).

Areas that are soft, loose, or 'wiggly' are unacceptable, even on extremely thin bodies. Cellulite management, like liposuction, has nothing to do with weight loss, and everything to do with the quest for firm bodily margins. (ibid.: 90)

We have, thus far, concentrated principally on diet as a way of regulating the size and shape of the body, as well as being an indicator of a personal morality: thin bodies represent controlled and cared-for bodies; fat bodies suggest some sort of moral failing. There are, however, other ways in which the body can be managed and sculptured. Surgical intervention, most commonly in the form of cosmetic surgery to alter appearance, is an obvious example. Parts of the body can be enlarged or changed in appearance, as in the practice of breast enhancement. Far more radical, however, is the case of gender realignment, or sex change. Complex surgical procedures, combined with the use of hormones and counselling, can help a person complete the transition from male to female or vice versa. The body, and in particular the genitalia, are the most obvious indicators of our sex. Paul Hewitt writes movingly of his own experiences as a female-to-male transsexual: 'It is not that I *want* to be male. I *am* male, and, like all transsexuals, I experience an overwhelming urge to bring the gender of my body into line with the gender of my mind' (Hewitt and Warren 1997: 75).

Changing his outward appearance allows him to pass as a man. Male dress, male haircuts and clothes all play an important part in signalling to others that he is male, but more fundamental changes are needed: the possession of an artificial penis and the removal of both breasts. This alone should be evidence that the body is *the* ultimate means of displaying who we are to others.

Question

Which new technologies have made us rethink our understanding of our bodies?

10.4 The 'failed' body: ill health and disease

We now continue these themes, but move on to an examination of the ways in which disability and chronic illness transform the body and personal identity.

Increasingly, most heavyweight newspapers carry a regular column written by someone with some form of chronic illness providing insights into their life and the challenges that chronic illness brings. Also, with the widening use of the internet, people with chronic illnesses set up and write their own blogs. These discuss various aspects of living with a variety of illnesses (Hardey 2002; Seale 2005). Many blogs or columns are written from an 'open secret' position, in that both writer and reader know that at some point the author may well die. Over the years we have seen columns and books dealing with, for example, HIV/AIDS (Oscar Moore with 'PWA' [People With AIDS]), breast cancer (Ruth Picardie with 'Before I say good-bye'). These glimpses into the life of someone with a long-term, probably fatal condition are deeply moving, and readers feel a strong sense of attachment to the writer. Such articles and serials are also indicative of how chronic illness is moving centre stage in terms of the general awareness of health and illness. Most people in the UK now will die of a chronic illness rather than from an infectious disease – many more than in previous centuries. The increase in the number of people with chronic illnesses raises several important issues:

- The dominance of medical science and its ability to cure all is challenged; its weaknesses and limits are exposed.
- The person with a chronic illness has to reconstruct aspects of their life and identity when facing a condition that will become a fundamental part of their existence.

We can see these concerns in this extract from Picardie (1993: 1), when she is corresponding with a friend about forthcoming treatment and her wider anxieties about her family:

The latest news is that I didn't have the second lot of chemo yesterday, because my white blood cell count is still crap – they went in 'all guns blazing' (direct quote from oncologist) first time round and it was obviously OTT .... Meanwhile, my hair is falling out with amazing rapidity – I estimate total baldness will be achieved by the weekend, so the whole thing will have happened in a week. It's getting awfully expensive – had my hair cut ultra short on Monday, and reckon I will have to have it shaved on Friday. I was a bit freaked out at first – it's really alarming running your hand through your hair and handfuls coming out. Makes you look sick, feel that you are dying, etc., which I am not .... Meanwhile, I am asking everyone I know to buy me a hat. I hope I don't frighten the children – I imagine I'll look pretty weird.

In this extract, Picardie records her ambivalence toward the chemotherapy treatment, which was, at that time, resulting only in hair loss. She is also battling to maintain 'normality' by seeking to minimise the impact and disruption that being bald may have on her children. These themes of identity and maintaining a 'normal life', will be explored in this section. Sociologists such as Anslem Strauss, Ilene Lubkin and Michael Bury have developed useful perspectives and ideas for understanding the many complexities and subtleties that surround people with chronic illnesses in contemporary western societies. Much research has focused on how people readapt their lives, organise resources and present themselves to the outside world.

In particular we will look at the work of Bury (1991) and the following concepts he has devised that help us sociologically explore chronic illness:

- biographical disruption
- adjusting to the impact of treatment regimens
- adaptation and management of illness

Before going any further, it should be emphasised that we are not looking at a formal model or stages that people go through as their lives with a chronic illness unfold. Rather, we are looking at issues that face them at various points during their lives. The various concepts listed above should be seen as *emergent* and not *sequential*. This means that there is no ordered 'timetable', as to how a condition develops over time and what symptoms a person with a chronic illness will experience and when they will experience them. For example, with multiple sclerosis people with the condition often have no idea how the illness will develop in their life. There is almost a 'randomness' in when symptoms appear or emerge and how they will have to respond to the changes that those symptoms bring to their life when they appear.

Biographical disruption

Biographical disruption refers to a destabilisation, questioning and reorganisation of identity after the onset of chronic illness.

Biographical disruption is a core concept in the sociological study of chronic illness, and has helped to illuminate and explore the lived experience of people with chronic illnesses (Williams 2000). In this section, we will look at what biographical disruption means and entails, as well as the subtleties and nuances that go along with it, before moving on to some of the criticisms that have been made.

First of all, let us turn to looking at what biographical disruption means as a concept. Think of your life as narrative, as a story that has been partially written with past events apparently well defined and recorded, the present unfolding, and the future a set of plans, ambitions and hopes. Now imagine that personal biography being radically altered as you learn that your body is failing, that cells are under attack or your brain is sending out a series of 'bizarre' signals that prevent your limbs functioning as they once did. Suddenly, all that narrative, that 'biography', you have constructed for yourself and hope to build for the future is thrown into doubt. The present now has to be renegotiated (worked out), the future seems doubtful and the past a strange place. In short, you have to face a disruption in your concept of self and in your 'own biography'. This is something that Charmaz (1983) has described as the 'loss of self', where you see your former self crumble and disappear. Frank (1995), too, has used similar dramatic language to capture an image of the wreckage of one's life following the onset of chronic illness.

Question

Think of your life as a narrative – What has been written so far and what have you plotted out for the future?

For someone with a chronic illness, biographical disruption often entails a reorganisation of their life on many levels; various ideas of self and of relationships with family, friends and colleagues will be challenged and re-evaluated. Within the biographical disruption of life the individual will have to deal with the *consequences* and *significance* of the illness (Bury 1997). We can see some of this, for example, in a study on multiple sclerosis (MS) by Boeije et al. (2002). They found that for the people in their research many parts of their lives, which they held to be important as part of their self-identity, had to be reconsidered. One useful example is that of Marc, a young man in his early thirties, who was dedicated to his job and was a keen windsurfer; an activity that was a key part of his social life (Boeije et al. 2002: 886). The changes in his body brought on by the MS meant that he was unable to go to work and to socialise as he had before the onset of the condition. To deal with these issues, he began to relish having free time, something he thought he would be unable to do and develop new hobbies with friends, such as playing cards. As Marc says:

> When I was working I was almost a workaholic. So I thought that I would go crazy sitting at home all day. But I still know how to enjoy things, it's wonderful having all these days off. Beforehand, you don't expect that to happen, but I've got such nice people around me and I often have visitors. That never seems to stop. I can open the doors with my remote control from my bedroom, which is ideal. I have contact with all kinds of people, including fellow sufferers. (Boeije et al. 2002: 886)

The actual symptoms of a condition will affect everyday life. Someone, for example, with temporal lobe epilepsy (or petit mal epilepsy as it was formerly called) may have to live with the uncertainty of not knowing when or in what context they may have an absence (Iphofen 1996). This can make certain social situations fraught with risk, in terms of safety or, more importantly, of breaking social norms. For other conditions, there are issues of self-care and managing symptoms on a daily basis. As mentioned in Chapter 1, illness also has cultural and metaphorical significance. People with chronic illness may have to respond to the way in which their culture and society perceive their condition. Certain conditions carry a social **stigma** when the illness is connected with undesirable states or social deviance. Younger people with arthritis feel that they are ageing prematurely (Singer 1974), while people with HIV/AIDS could be stigmatised as 'junkies', given the association of HIV/AIDS with substance use, for example. It is important to note here that it is not the person with chronic illness that is 'the problem', but rather societal attitudes and the way in which the physical environment is shaped. We will explore this highly important and fundamental issue later in this chapter, when we look at disability.

There has been some debate surrounding the assumption that biography is always disrupted after the onset of a chronic illness. Pound et al. (1998) have argued that for older people development of a chronic illness (stroke, in their research) was in some ways expected and regarded as a 'normal crisis'. The impact of the stroke, and the consequent disruption of biography, was lessened by the fact that it was just one of many 'disruptive' issues (such as poverty and poor housing) that faced this group of people. Faircloth et al. (2004) also explored this idea of age and other factors in studying how people could minimise biographical disruption. In their study, also on stroke, they too found that age reduced the disruptive effects of stroke on older people's understandings and perceptions of who they were and their wider identity. They also found that the presence, and a history, of other illnesses (such as diabetes) and knowledge of stroke (typically seeing it happen to other people) also helped people who had experienced a stroke view it as a normal part of life. Thus, they were better set to handle the changes in their lives that having a stroke entailed. To some extent having a stroke was part of the 'biographical flow', where chronic illness was just part of the rhythms and expectations of everyday life, especially, in this case, for older people.

Schnittker (2005) noted that age could act as a factor in lessening disruption for someone with a chronic illness generally. He found that depression as a consequence of chronic illness seemed more likely to affect people who had become chronically ill when younger rather than those who had become chronically ill when they were older. This was possibly due to older people having developed more complex emotional skills over their **life course**, which could help them cope with illness.

Reviewing the literature on biographical disruption, Williams (2000) has offered further refinements to this core concept. Following Pound et al. (1998), he suggested that chronic illness cannot be seen exclusively as *disruption* but could be viewed as *continuity*, where chronic illness is expected and regarded as normal due to age and class. In the case of gay men with HIV/AIDS, for instance, the onset of infection or the development of non-symptomatic HIV can also lead to an affirmation of political identity, something that Carricaburu and Pierret (1995) describe as 'biographical reinforcement'. Williams cites other examples, too numerous to mention here, but all with the same theme – that the context of someone's life has a strong bearing on how disruptive a chronic illness will be.

Question

Discuss the concept of biographical disruption. How accurate do you think it is in exploring the experiences of people with chronic conditions?

Impact of treatment regimens

One major adjustment that inevitably comes with a chronic illness is incorporating medical and clinical treatments into daily life. We will look here at how treatment regimens can impact on a person with a chronic illness and also why people with a chronic illness do not always go along with what they are told to do by medical experts and therapists. A key point here is that what a health professional thinks is the best form of treatment or therapy may not be accepted by someone with a chronic illness for a whole host of complex, but legitimate, reasons as the best way forward. For example, someone with MS may be encouraged by a therapist to use a wheelchair. This may be a sensible course of action from the therapist's perspective, as it allows the person with MS a degree of mobility that they may not currently have. For the person with MS, however, a wheelchair may signify a massive change in their life, both on a symbolic and a personal level, with using a wheelchair being a very strong indicator that they are becoming a disabled person and are no longer the person they once perceived themselves as being.

There are two main ways in which treatment regimens impact on people with a chronic illness. Treatment regimens that are part and parcel of living with chronic illness vary widely both in the form they take (for example, having to use a stoma, having regular dialysis or taking a variety of medication) and in the impact that they may have (more of which later). Such impacts can be either *affective* (to do with people's emotions and how they see themselves), or *instrumental* (reorganising time and learning to manage technology and medication), though they both, to a great extent, overlap.

If we look at *affective* changes first of all, what we see is that treatment can alter how you think about yourself both in relation to your past biography and in relation to other people – particularly, if the treatment has potentially stigmatising consequences. MacDonald (1988), for example, observed that for people with a colostomy, following treatment for rectal cancer, there was a strong tendency to conceal information about their stoma. The patients felt that the odours, noise and dealing with the bag in public places were potentially disruptive to normal social intercourse. These patients with rectal cancer were further stigmatised in a variety of ways. In addition to having to negotiate the stigma of cancer, they also broke cultural taboos concerning faeces and their disposal. As a result, social situations became fraught with risk, with patients seeking to minimise the impact of the stigma, fearing embarrassment or disgust. Overall, for these patients, there was some impairment of quality of life, even if they had managed to deal with the socially perceived 'problems' of their stomas in some way.

While involved in long-term treatment or therapy there exists the problem of what Robinson (1988) terms the 'medical merry-go-round'. Here the person with a chronic illness experiences their expectations, and emotional highs and lows, of what treatment will deliver going up and down as they circle through various forms and stages of treatment or medication, in a way that is similar to an old-fashioned carousel ride where the horses go up and down and continually move in a circle. This can be very emotionally and physically draining and exhausting. Research by Wiles et al. (2004) provides a useful example of this. Looking at people who were undergoing physiotherapy after a stroke, Wiles et al. found that clients had to manage feelings of potential disappointment when their time with the physiotherapist was at an end. Though the patients usually felt disappointment at no longer receiving 'physio' they often left with high expectations that their future recovery was going to continue and overall function improve – something that, given the uncertainties of stroke recovery, may be unlikely to happen. Wiles et al. (2004) draw attention to the need for therapists to be wary of the emotional aspects of a client's therapy as part of the therapy process, as well as how to manage feelings of optimism and disappointment.

If we turn now to the *instrumental* effects of treatment regimens we can see that compliance/adherence to medication, meeting the demands of clinical appointments and using medical technology can also be very complex. Compliance/adherence to medication used to be regarded as almost a straightforward example of medicalisation within medical sociology, where the medical world took over another part of someone's private life-world. There has been a shift lately, however, in thinking about how people with chronic conditions relate to medication. Instead of being seen in 'black-and-white' terms, of people meekly following what they are told, people are seen as thoughtfully engaging with the medication as part of their wider adjustments to changes in the self brought about by chronic illness.

This means that it is not a simple case of the medical expert giving out advice or instructing someone in what to do and that person going meekly along with what they have been told. Such, an idea is evident in Parsons' idea of the sick role, which is discussed in Chapter 3. Increasingly, as Pound et al. (2005) note, people adopt a strategic position on medication and treatment, whereby they will often see how well treatment regimens work in the context of their lives before deciding whether or not to comply. As a result health professionals have to develop more flexible and fluid ways of interacting, adopting a variety of roles and approaches to encourage people with chronic illnesses to engage with and adopt certain treatment regimens. This may entail health professionals acting as 'educators, detectives, negotiators, salesmen, cheerleaders and policemen' (Lutfey 2005: 421), when working with clients.

Adaptation and management of illness

From the discussion so far, we see that chronic illness can have a considerable impact on your life. Aspects of your life may be thrown into question and have to be re-evaluated, while the treatment for the condition can produce a whole host of potentially stigmatising situations. Within this context people with chronic illnesses nevertheless seek to maintain some sense of self and identity. In the earlier quote from Picardie there was evidence of how she dealt with hair loss by having her hair cut short in an attempt to appear 'normal'. Bury (1991) describes these responses as coping, strategy and style:

- *Coping* is a term used in a variety of contexts, commonly when someone is coping with the illness, whether successfully or not. It can also take on emotional dimensions and relate to how someone is holding on to certain aspects of identity.
- *Strategy* is the particular actions or resources someone utilises to deal with problems created by the illness and by social responses. They can range from breaking the day down into manageable chunks to avoiding the general public to minimise the risk of stigma.
- *Style* is how one presents oneself to the social world in an attempt to maintain aspects of self.

10.5 Disabled people and disability

One of the potential consequences of chronic illness is a disability of some kind. Many of the conditions mentioned in the previous section can lead to some level of impaired function or changes in how the body operates in particular contexts. This section will explore issues of disability in general and in relation to chronic illness.

The first point to consider is what we actually mean by disability. Common images of disability often show people in wheelchairs, images that are overlain with notions of dependency, weakness, misfortune and charity. As we have seen elsewhere in this book, there is no such thing as a neutral expression and all aspects of terminology and imagery are cultural products often reflecting issues concerning power and regulation. Disability is no exception, and in attempting to study disability, analysing and looking at what concepts lie behind various terms is a useful introduction. The following terms circulate in lay **discourse** about people with disabilities:

- cripple/crippled
- the handicapped
- deformed
- 'something wrong'
- the disabled

They may all appear to be quite separate terms, some more acceptable (the disabled) than others (cripple). However, underneath them all there is the same negative attitude towards people with impaired or disabled bodies. They all remove the person from the experience of disability and frame disability in terms of mechanical body parts gone 'wrong'. Terms such as '*the* disabled' and '*the* handicapped' imply that there is no person there, simply a medical condition with no personal narrative, identity or desires. Moreover, such expressions imply that everyone who is disabled has a uniform experience regardless of gender, class, **ethnicity**, age, sexuality or impairment. There is also a very negative history connected to the word 'handicapped'. The term originates in the medieval expression to go 'cap in hand' or to beg. This carries the implication that people with disabilities occupy an inferior position in society as outsiders reliant upon charity and incapable of independently supporting themselves.

Question

What terms for disability do you find acceptable and why?

We have discussed certain negative words and expressions used in connection with disability. There are other expressions that avoid some of these pitfalls. Indeed, they have been used already in this text: people with disabilities or disabled people. Both terms avoid medicalising people's existence, and also emphasise the person with their range of differences, emotions and identity. However, we can still question the language a little further – what do terms such as 'impairment' and 'disability' mean? Here we find another area of controversy. The following definition of impairment, disability and handicap was used by the World Health Organisation (1980) until quite recently:

Impairment
Any loss or abnormality, of physiological or anatomical structure or function. Thus impairment could range from a scar on the skin to a malfunction of the liver or heart.

Disability
Any restriction or lack of ability to perform an activity, as a result of impairment, in a manner or within the range considered normal for a human being, for example the ability to climb the stairs or walk to the shops.

Handicap
A disadvantage for a given individual, resulting from an impairment or a disability, that limits or prevents the fulfilment of a role for that individual (depending on such factors as age, sex and social and cultural factors). Handicap refers to the disadvantage the individual encounters, as a result of the impairment and/or disability, when compared with his or her peers.

This particular definition has been heavily criticised for its strong medical orientation and for placing the source of disability in the individual rather than in wider factors. It also contains the implication that, by not being able, because of impairment, to carry out an activity considered normal, a person with a disability must therefore be *abnormal*. As writers such as Oliver (1990) note, the WHO definition follows a non-disabled person's view of disability, thus failing to understand or comprehend the full experience of someone with a disability. The model implies that it is the disabled person who must adjust and adapt to the world, because it is they who are problematic and not the arrangement of built spaces or social attitudes (Barnes et al. 1999).

Compare that definition with those proposed by Finkelstein and French:

Impairment
Impairment is the lack of part or all of a limb, or having a defective limb, organ or mechanism of the body.

Disability
Disability is the loss or limitation of opportunities that prevents people who have impairments from taking part in the normal life of the community on an equal level with others due to physical and social barriers. (Finkelstein and French 1993: 28)

This is substantially different from the first definition we looked at. Here the emphasis is on societal factors such as the design of buildings or discriminatory attitudes of others, a far cry from regarding an individual's body as the cause of disability.

At the heart of this discussion is how we see or define disability. There is a range of models that various writers propose, but two models stand out in particular when it comes to conceptualising disability: the medical model and the social model:

- The **medical model** of disability has a strong emphasis on seeing disability as an individual tragedy where, by a quirk of fate either genetic or accidental, someone becomes disabled and their life is, in many ways, ruined. They are incapable of functioning in a productive manner and without the assistance, help and intervention of certain highly trained specialists their lives would be almost impossible. As a result, power and decision making is in the hands of the professionals. Physical dysfunction and the failure of body parts are emphasised in this approach, which strongly focuses on disability as due to the person, with other factors being ignored. This model is implicitly negative in its depiction of disabled people.
- The **social model** of disability argues that prejudicial attitudes, disabling environments and cultural barriers socially create disability. The focus here is on self-help and emancipation, as it calls for civil rights and for disabled people themselves to be empowered to make decisions about what support and services they receive. Disabled people are also more than capable of leading fulfilling lives that are productive, rewarding or as fraught with problems as those of non-disabled people, and disability is no bar to sexuality. Ultimately, disability is a mixture of factors that includes impairments as well as cultural, social, material and attitudinal factors. This model is implicitly positive in its portrayal of people with disabilities.

Question

Which of the above models do you think your particular health profession follows? Did you find anything challenging in how you conceptualize disability in light of what you have read about the medical model or the social model?

Links

Chapters 2 and 3 discuss other aspects of client–professional interactions.

The medical profession and para-professions, such as occupational therapy and physiotherapy, have been criticised for following the medical model, whether intentionally or not (French 1994; Johnson 1993; Stalker and Jones 1998). Therapists or doctors often take the lead in therapeutic encounters, with the professional dominating the decision making on the grounds that they 'know best':

> the attitudes of physiotherapists were often perceived as patronising and undermining. . . . Prescriptive labelling and treatment of people according to impairment was seen as a denial of individuality and typical of therapist centred physiotherapy.
> (Johnson 1993: 624)

This is the main challenge of the **social model of disability**: that all health professionals, not just physiotherapists, must change or reflect upon how they practise. Even though they may perceive themselves as losing power and overall control, they should defer more to the needs of the disabled person with whom they are working.

Question

How do those last comments make you feel? Do you think that health professionals may not be as holistic as they portray themselves to be?

The sociology of the body draws attention to two concepts of the body: the body as *Körper* and the body as *Leib* (Shilling 1993). '*Körper*' refers to the body as 'the objective, exterior, institutionalised body' (Williams and Bendelow 1998). This way of viewing the body is evident when anatomy or physiology is studied. The body is presented as a series of structures and constructions that can be described as objects that are without emotions and that are not seen as being part of a person. In many ways this is how medicalised views of disability operate. The disabled individual is not seen as a disabled *person* but as a *body* that has something wrong with it and, therefore, as something that can be 'fixed' or repaired. Moreover, as Edwards (1998) argues, seeing the body as a separate objective entity can make understanding disability difficult.

He cites the work of Wendell who explores her experiences of ME (myalgic encephalomyelitis) (1996: 21–2) and her problems of trying to express the psychological and physical aspects of disability as not being separate.

'*Leib*' refers to the body as 'the animated, living, experiential body' (Williams and Bendelow 1998). Here the body is seen in an embodied context whereby the body and mind form the same entity and all aspects of the physical body, the emotions and personal narrative form one whole. This perspective, which allows us to see the body and the self as one, could overcome the problems of trying to conceptualise and explore the lived experience of disability, or as Overboe (1999: 24) puts it when discussing disability in this context: 'Thus our "lived experience" would be an integral part of the atmosphere and atone for any change within our lives and our interaction with others, whether they be disabled or non-disabled.'

Focusing on the *Leib* experience can help us understand the emergent characteristics of disability and identity. Following this approach, Williams and Barlow's (1998) study of arthritis identified that body and mind, the embodied lived experience, were not separate. Subjects reported how feelings of self and identity emerged through the changes in their bodies. The women with arthritis felt themselves less attractive and feared that they were breaking a social taboo by displaying a 'pained' body in public. The influence of consumerism and notions of the body perfect were at play here, with the women feeling that they did not accord with these images.

Conclusion

This chapter has shown that the human body is not just a biological entity but is inextricably bound up with society, culture and history. Much of how we project our identity and develop a sense of self that is important and vital in our everyday interactions is performed through and with our bodies. This use of the body is becoming more central in the consumerist society in which we live, where a thin, toned body adorned in the most current of fashion styles is presented as being highly desirable. Television shows, magazines and commercials extol the supposed virtues of such an appearance. Obviously, only a very few people (usually celebrities with financial and other resources) can obtain that look and the pressure to conform to such appearances can result in misery and suffering for many people.

The importance of the body in identity is brought into sharp relief in relation to chronic illness. Here, the emergence of symptoms and changes in the body disrupts the sense of self and can challenge how we see our lives. This can lead to all sorts of re-evaluations of identity and how to lead a life with the destabilization that chronic illness can bring. This 'pessimistic' take on chronic illness should, however, be tempered by research that indicates that sometimes chronic illness is 'not that bad'. Age and class, for example, can provide an emotional resilience and acceptance of chronic illness.

The body and identity are also visible in disability issues. Sociological perspectives focus on disability as the outcome of prejudicial and discriminatory social attitudes and perceptions. Bodies that do not match or that are 'different' from an able-bodied norm are devalued, and disabled people's identities are given a lesser social status. Disabled people have advanced a civil rights agenda to counteract many of the negative and oppressive structures that act against them being fairly treated in society.

SUMMARY POINTS

- The taken-for-granted status of the body has detracted from the significance of the body for students of the sociology of health.
- Human experiences are essentially embodied and this is most true of health and illness.
- The body is a bearer of values and a means of representing our identity to others.
- The civilised body is one that is controlled both in terms of bodily functions and displays of emotion.
- The limits of the physical body are constantly being extended as scientific advances allow us to alter the appearance of our bodies and to replace diseased organs.
- Ideas about the body are underpinned by normative concepts of the 'good' and 'bad' body, the former being associated with bodily perfection.
- Any form of disease, but particularly chronic and terminal conditions, bring into stark reality the limits and fallibility of the human body.
- A 'failed' body forces individuals to reassess their lives and sense of identity – though this is not necessarily a negative experience.
- Disability is a combination of environmental, social, cultural, material and physical factors. Acknowledging disability in this way asks fundamental questions of health professionals when interacting with disabled people.

Case study

Consider the following case study and then answer the questions below.

James was diagnosed with rheumatoid arthritis around the time of his eighth birthday. The condition has meant that at times his mobility has been severely affected. Games and sports at school were something that he had to miss out on. Writing for long periods in exams became impossible in his final year and so he produced his work on a laptop in a room separate from the rest of his classmates. After finishing school, James wanted to enter a career in hotel management but this proved impossible as the type of work involved a considerable amount of time spent on one's feet, something James could not do without being in severe pain. Instead, he chose a clerical post in the Civil Service which would allow him to be seated for much of the day and to use a PC instead of physically writing.

1 Mobility was a problem for James from an early age. What kinds of activities and experiences do you

think that he might have missed out on compared to other children his age?

2   How might you apply the concept of 'biographical disruption' to James' experiences as a young adult?

3   What kind of knowledge would you have expected James to accumulate about this condition? How would this differ from the knowledge of the clinician and what, if any, would be its relevance to anyone treating James?

Taking your studies further

This chapter will have helped you understand many of the key terms, concepts, theories and debates relating to the body. Listed below are journal articles and books that will provide deeper and more detailed discussions of the points raised in this chapter. You will also find what is available on the companion website. This offers downloads of relevant material, plus links to useful websites in addition to podcasts and other features.

Recommended reading

Books and chapters

Barnes, C. and Mercer, G. (2003) *Disability*. Cambridge: Polity.

Bordo, S. (1990) 'Reading the slender body', in M. Jacobs, E.F. Keller and S. Shuttleworth (eds), *Body/Politics: Women and the Discourse of Science*. New York: Routledge.

Bury, M. (1997) *Health and Illness in a Changing Society*. London: Routledge.

Hawkes, G. (1996) *A Sociology of Sex and Sexuality*. Buckingham: Open University Press.

Hockey, J. and James, A. (2007) *Embodying Health Identities*. Basingstoke: Palgrave Macmillan.

Shilling, C. (2003) *The Body and Social Theory*, 2nd edn. London: SAGE.

Shilling, C. (2007) *Embodying Sociology: Retrospect, Progress and Prospects*. Oxford: Blackwell.

Williams, S.J., Bendelow, G. and Birke, L. (2003) *Debating Biology: Sociological Reflections on Health, Medicine and Society*. London: Routledge.

Journal articles

Bury, M (2001) 'Illness narratives: fact or fiction?' *Sociology of Health and Illness*, 23 (3): 263–85.

Pound, P. Gompertz, P. and Ebrahim, S. (1998) 'Illness in the context of older age: the case of stroke,' *Sociology of Health and Illness*, 20 (4): 489–506.

On the companion website

Frank, A.W. (1997) 'Illness as moral occasion: restoring agency to ill people', *Health*, 4 (1): 131–48.

Williams, S.J. (2003) *Medicine and the Body*. London: SAGE, Chapter 5.

11

Health, ageing and the life course

MAIN POINTS

- Old age and ill health are not synonymous, with the majority of older people living fit, healthy and active lives.
- Older people can be subject to ageist stereotyping and this can impact on identity and sense of self.
- It is important to understand ageing as taking place in biographical and historical time. Experiences across the life course strongly influence the health of older people.

KEY CONCEPTS

Ageism, attitudes, Third Age, life course, biographical and historical time, the body.

Introduction

Throughout Europe and North America more and more people are living into old age as the post-war baby boom generation reaches that phase of their lives. In the UK, for example, in 1951 there were 13.8 million people over the age of 50; this compares to 20 million over 50 in 2003 (ONS 2005a: 1). Figure 11.1 displays other important and significant ways in which the age composition of the older population has changed in the UK comparing 1951 to 2003 and projecting ahead to 2031. This increase in the number of older people in **society** is visible in developing nations too, with the United Nations predicting that by 2050 older people will comprise 20 per cent of the population in developing regions. This demographic shift raises many interesting issues and challenges both for society and for the sociological study of what it means to be an older person. As will be explored in this chapter, being older is not a simple case of having grey hair, worsening health and living alone, as popular stereotypes sometimes hold; it is a complex mix of lifestyles, social perceptions and levels of health.

11.1 Ageing in society: a general overview

The body begins to age, change and develop from the moment of birth until its eventual death. This, though, should not be read as meaning that ageing is purely a biological phenomenon driven entirely by the alterations to the surface layers of skin and hair paralleled by decreasing mental acuity and all-round physiological decline. Rather, ageing, as a phase of one's life, is the product of three factors that all weave together: biology, psychology and the social. Each of these factors can exert an influence on the others. So, for example, going grey may be a physical sign of ageing in some sense, but it depends on the society of which one is a member whether having grey hair means someone is deemed to be 'old' and should be treated in a different way from someone who does not have grey hair. It is through the social that experiences, perceptions and attitudes to what it is to be old and what is regarded as being old are mediated and created. Similarly, a society can exert such pressure and stress on someone that this hastens their biological ageing. Among the more overt social aspects of ageing in society are certain negative attitudes expressed by individuals. It is to a discussion of '**ageism**' that attention turns to next.

Ageism

In other chapters we have looked at other forms of **discrimination** and **prejudice** in the form of sexism and **racism**. We saw how socially created perceptions of people's characteristics (their **sex** or **ethnicity**) act as barriers that prevent women and

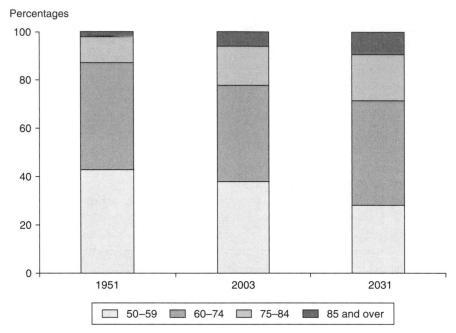

Percentages

FIGURE 11.1   *Age composition of the older population, UK (ONS 2003a)*
Source: National Statistics Website: www.statistics.gov.uk
Crown copyright material is reproduced with the permission of the Controller of HMSO
Reproduced under the terms of the Click-Use License

people from ethnic minority groups having a full and equal place in society. Such barriers can have a negative and harmful effect on their health. Ageism is yet another example of the many prejudices that exist within society. In popular culture there are many examples of this stereotype. A useful example is, arguably, Abe Simpson, the grandpa character in *The Simpsons*. In the episodes in which Abe appears the comedy content is generated by Abe falling asleep at inopportune moments or embarking on long rambling stories about his youth. Instances such as these match popular stereotypes that all old people are 'demented' and in poor health.

Defining Ageism:

1   A set of beliefs originating in biological variation related to the ageing process
2   The actions of corporate bodies and their agents, the resulting views of ordinary people.

> In consequence of this, it follows that:
>
> (a) Ageism generates and reinforces a fear and denigration of the ageing process, and stereotyping presumptions regarding competence and the need for protection.
> (b) In particular, ageism legitimates the use of chronological age to mark out classes of people who are systematically denied resources and opportunities that others enjoy, and who suffer the consequences of such denigration, ranging from well-meaning patronage to unambiguous vilification. (Bytheway and Johnson 1990 cited in Bytheway 1995: 14)

Ageism is, however, more than just finding old people amusing. It can take many other forms as well. At its worst it can be structurally located and act as a barrier to older people receiving appropriate health care. Age Concern England (2002) has noted the presence of two forms of ageism within the NHS. The first form is *direct ageism*, instances when actual policy or guidelines prevents someone from receiving appropriate health care based directly on their age. This is a very overt and easy to identify form of discrimination. The other form of ageism, *indirect ageism*, is more subtle and is concerned with attitudes and assumptions that the health of older people is less important than that of younger people.

Question

Identify positive and negative portrayals of older people in society. Which type of image is more frequently visible? Why do you think there is prejudice and discrimination against old people in current society?

11.2 Bodies and ageing

Despite the fact that this is the fate of us all, old age is often associated with negative images and attitudes. The earlier discussion of the sociology of the body illustrated the importance of our physical self for our sense of identity, and from this it is possible to see that the visible signs of ageing (greying hair and developing wrinkles, for example) act as a set of symbols, which can be read in often prejudicial and negative ways in society. This is especially so in a consumer society where an old body is often perceived as a less socially valued and acceptable body than a young fit, fat-free and athletic body. Indeed, the ever increasing range of cosmetics offering to hold back the onset of the signs of ageing is another way in which both the body is commodified (essentially one is compelled to purchase a youthful face and body) and youth is prioritised. Youth is clearly associated with notions of optimum physical performance (hence sports people are 'old' in their mid-thirties), cognitive ability and attractiveness. In contrast, old age is seen as a period of decline marked, for example, by loss of height and by wrinkled skin. This social impulse to maintain youth is especially problematic for women who, unlike men, are likely to be judged on their physical appearance – their looks – rather on any other criteria.

The continuing importance of the body and images of ageing can also be seen in the next example. One of the most important activities that we do with our bodies is to dress and present it with clothes that accord with what we wish to say about ourselves and what we believe to be socially appropriate. This can be a difficult balancing act at any stage of one's life, given the strong pressure to meet certain consumerist and cultural expectations. There are, though, certain issues that older people have to negotiate when they choose what to wear. Twigg (2007) draws our attention to how clothing is 'age-ordered', with certain styles of clothes deemed both age appropriate and a signifier of age. In some respects, this can be seen as an informal policing of how older people (women in particular) present themselves as they grow older. Often this means a toning down of style and opting for less 'flamboyant' styles. Twigg (2007: 296) uses an example from research by Holland (2004) to illustrate this point. Here, women who have an alternative style of dress (for example, grunge and Gothic styles involving dreadlocks, piercings and tattoos) indicated a sense of apprehension about having to alter their appearance as they grew older. The women in this study were worried that their alternative stylistic difference, which was an important part of their youthful identity, would be seen as being 'grotesque' if they maintained it into their middle years and beyond. The two phrases that sum up the association between youth, attractiveness and age are 'growing old gracefully' and 'mutton dressed as lamb' (Fairhurst 1998: 261). Both phrases make assumptions about age-appropriate actions and appearance. Mutton is older, tougher meat than youthful and tender lamb. Fairhurst's respondents all interpreted 'mutton dressed as lamb' as the wearing of 'inappropriate clothes, hair, make-up or jewellery' (ibid.: 262).

Featherstone and Hepworth (1993) also draw our attention to the largely negative terms used to describe older people. Such words include 'wrinkly', 'gaga', 'biddy', 'fogey' and 'geriatric' (1993: 308). The biological process of ageing is 'shaped or constructed in terms of symbolic imagery, both verbal and non verbal' (ibid.:). Words and images are used as stereotypes to make sense of and describe the experiences of older people. The danger of such stereotypes is that they fail to reflect the complexity and diversity of people's experiences of ageing.

These negative images of old age can permeate all aspects of ageing in society. One of the most common stereotypes is that old age is synonymous with decline and depedency; and that ageing is *itself* a disease or illness. These assumptions provide a useful starting point for a discussion of the assumed association between old age and ill health. As we will go on to discuss, many older people, on the contrary, enjoy a life relatively free from sickness and dependency. The same negative stereotyping of individuals on the basis of sickness and dependency can, arguably, be seen in relation to people with disabilities. Such an association may, therefore, lead us to conclude that it is the assumption of dependency and of an inability to perform socially that is the source of the discrimination rather than the actual age of the person.

Thus far we have given consideration to images of old age. The following section is concerned with placing those images within a theoretical context. The aim of this discussion is to illustrate through a sociological **analysis** that, much more than simply a physiological experience, age is fundamentally a social experience.

11.3 Sociological theories of ageing

Links

Disengagement theory is closely related to the functionalist perspective outlined in Chapter 1.

Sociology offers a number of perspectives, all of which seek to explain the social situation, status and role of older people. **Disengagement theory** offers what might appear in the twenty-first century a rather dated perspective on ageing and the role of older people. Cumming and Henry (1961) suggested that as people reach old age they gradually disengage from society, in terms of their social contacts, roles and responsibilities. The process of disengagement prepares the older person and society in general for the ultimate disengagement in the form of death or incapacity (Bond et al. 1993: 32). Disengagement theory is based on a broader functionalist perspective of society with its emphasis on the roles, responsibilities and values that ensure the smooth running of the social **structure**. By disengaging, for example through retirement from the paid workforce, individuals cease to be essential to the functioning of the social structure. On this basis their death does not result in any significant disruption since older people have ceased to be part of the workforce.

Bond et al. (1993) highlight a number of problems with this perspective on ageing. They argue, first, that disengagement theory condones the social isolation and marginalisation of older people, which for many results in poverty and loneliness. Second, they suggest that this **theory** is based on an assumption that disengagement is a natural and inevitable occurrence. It is possible to argue that the theory is essentially ageist in the sense that it assumes identical experiences for all older people. However, as Bond et al. (1993: 32) point out, many older people may still be actively engaged in society,

Disengagement theory states that older people relinquish their roles in society so as to minimise social disruption as they approach their final years. **Dependency theory** claims that older people's lives are restricted by poverty and not being able to access social and cultural resources. **Third age theory** points to old age as being a 'golden age' where enriching and rewarding experiences are available due to freedom from family and work commitments mediated by a consumerist society.

while for others old age is part of a lifelong experience of non-engagement and social isolation. The final criticism that can be made of disengagement theory is its failure to appreciate that certain social practices (such as enforced retirement from the paid workforce) and cultural values (ageism) combine to ensure that disengagement does become the experience of many older people. In this sense, we can perhaps appreciate that disengagement is the consequence of a specific set of social arrangements rather than a natural and inevitable part of the experience of ageing.

In contrast to disengagement theory, an alternative explanation of the experience of older people centres on the social creation of dependency. The essence of this approach is that older people are constructed as dependent on the state, primarily through exclusion from the paid workforce. Such exclusion also means that older people are further isolated from a wide variety of social settings, relationships and networks. Data indicates that older people are one of the groups most at risk of poverty because of their dependence largely on welfare benefits. The potential effects of retirement are, according to Bond et al. (1993: 34), poverty and restricted 'access to social resources in the form of a reduction in social relationships'.

So far, the discussion has focussed on what may be seen as pessimistic perspectives on ageing. We shall now turn to what might be regarded as more optimistic perspectives; where growing older opens up the possibilities of a phase in one's life that is filled with rich and rewarding experiences, free of the binds of work and other commitments. Such perspectives also draw our attention to some of the complexities of growing older in contemporary society, brought about by changes in welfare provision and the all-pervasive influence of consumer culture offering a range of possibilities on *how* to be an older person. Here, older people are seen to have more freedom to choose and decide their own identities and lifestyles.

Key to this more optimistic perspective is the work of Laslett (1987, 1989) and his concept of the 'Third Age'. He is calling for a reworking of how society views the different stages of moving through life. Essentially, the 'Third Age' involves a transition from various states of dependence to independence and from responsibility to increasing freedom and flexibility. So, the 'First Age' is childhood, when we are dependent on our parents, the 'Second Age' is the independence of being a mature person and being able to provide for yourself but perhaps 'hemmed' in by responsibilities of raising a family and holding down a job. The 'Third Age' is a period of life between later middle age and early older age. It is marked by increasing freedom from the constraints of work and family concerns, and can also be a 'golden age' occupied with activities that lead to a sense of fulfilment, self-realisation and personal growth. More recently, Laslett (1996) has added a 'Fourth Age', where physical decline and health problems begin to dominate the experiences of people in deeper old age, that is those above the age of 75.

The Third Age has been made possible by the increasing numbers, affluence and health of older people. This, combined with a consumer culture, which blurs many of the distinctions between the age groups, has allowed older people to escape the social expectations of how they should lead their lives and to strike out and create identities of their own.

There are, however, criticisms of this approach. For example, Bury (2000) has raised objections that the research is 'data light', meaning that more research has to be carried out to see if this 'Third Age' is actually happening, or whether it is more of an idea of what could happen given the changes indicated above. Another criticism is that this phase of self-realisation after one has retired is only open to those with the financial means to do so. One could argue that poverty still affects the lives of many older people, thus effectively preventing them from engaging in the consumerist activities that are so much part of the 'Third Age'. Just over 20 per cent of pensioners are living in poverty (ONS 2005a), though this is worse for older people from ethnic minority backgrounds and people in deeper old age.

Question

Which theory do you find the most persuasive and why?

11.4 Health and the life course

As was outlined above, there is often an almost taken-for-granted association between ageing, disability and ill health. The reality is far different from that with many older people living healthy active lives, especially for the 'younger' old. Table 11.1 indicates that many older people remain free of any long-standing illness or disability. For example, while just over 47 per cent of women aged between 65 and 84 did report a long-standing illness or disability, just under 53 per cent did not and, one can assume, enjoyed reasonable health (ONS 2005a). A closer examination of these figures does, however, reveal some subtle but important differences. In terms of **gender**, older women experience more health problems than men of the same age. It is also clear that some distinction should be made between age groups within the catch-all category of old age. Field (1992) draws a distinction between the 'young old' and the 'old old', the former below 75 and the latter over 85. Although the cut-off points might seem a little arbitrary, they are, nevertheless, helpful in identifying a trend towards increased levels of disability and ill health among older people over the age of 75 (Field 1992: 276).

Being old is simply – and obviously – not just always having been a certain age for all one's life. Older age is just another of the many elements and phases that go to make up your life. How that life is lived, however, greatly influences health in the older years, both in terms of developing, for example, long-term illness or a disability, and also shaping how illness and health is experienced and perceived. A useful concept in trying to understand this relationship between health and old age is that of the **life course**

Table 11.1   *Older people reporting a limiting long-term illness: by age and sex, 2001 England and Wales (Percentages) (ONS 2005b)*

	50–54	55–59	60–64	65–74	75–84	85 and over
Men	19.9	26.7	37.4	42.9	56	70.2
Women	21.1	27.5	32.1	40.6	58.9	78.3

Source: ONS (2005b)
Crown copyright material is reproduced with the permission of the Controller of HMSO
Reproduced under the terms of the Click-Use Licence

Life cycle is a concept borrowed from natural science and implies a series of set rigid stages that humans move through in their lives. **Life course** as a concept points to the increasing fluidity and fragmentation of contemporary society and reflects the fact that old certainties of what one does at certain points in one's life are increasingly unstable.

(Hockey and James 2003). In the past, moving through life was conceptualised as being similar to a cycle and commonly expressed using the term **life cycle**. Aspects of moving through life in this context were seen as inescapable certainties in life encountered by every generation. This included such events as school, work, marriage and starting a family. Overall, life-cycle approaches conceive life as being a set of rigid stages that one goes through without any variance or personal choice. In contrast, life in this current phase of modernity has become increasingly complex, fluid and fragmented. The certainties that are implied in a life-cycle approach are no longer with us and there can exist great varieties in how people experience and choose to live their lives. So, for example, people increasingly do not always enter into marriage or may delay having children, if they make that decision at all. By seeing life as a *course* that one takes through life where one has a certain latitude in making choices, rather than a *cycle* over which one has little control, such variety can be easier to understand.

Regarding ageing in context of both 'biographical' and 'historical' time is important to the life-course approach. (Bury 2000). Biographical time refers to the personal events in your life; for example, developing relationships, or choosing to go travelling, or what you did at university. Historical time refers to the events and social attitudes that mark particular phases in history; for example, the Second World War, or the changes in attitudes towards sexuality that took place in the 1960s. Though biographical time and historical time may seem quite different, they do relate to each other. Historical time can set the scene for what happens and unfolds in biographical time, giving a particular generation a shared set of beliefs and common experiences.

Question

Sketch out your life course so far. Identify both your biographical time and the historical time in which you live. What aspects of historical time help shape the identity of your generation?

Thinking of ageing in this way helps us to understand older people's health in two main ways. First, acknowledging a biographical element allows us to see that not all older people are a homogeneous social group and alike in all manner of ways. Rather, it draws attention to the importance of difference and how people can age in the same historical time but do so in their own individual way and how events in their past affect their health in the present. Second, the historical element can help us understand that people are part of a particular generation and how the experience of being part of that generation (this is called a *cohort effect*) shapes their health beliefs and attitudes towards illness. Ultimately though, it is the human body on which the experiences of both biographical and historical time will be 'recorded' in terms of good or bad health in older age. Blane et al. (2004: 2171) usefully summarise this point:

> The body can be seen as a mechanism which stores the past benefits and dis-benefits to which it has been exposed, either because damage at a critical period of development causes irreparable loss or because the effects of various types of damage accumulate over time.

So, for example, coming from a deprived background in childhood and working in an occupation that was tightly supervised and low in control could lead to poor health for an older person. Conversely, the opposite – material stability and an enjoyable career – is much more likely to mean good health for an older person. These are themes that we have explored in other chapters and that indicate, once more, how social influences, such as **class**, strongly influence health. Berney et al. (2000), for instance, found that both negative material and psycho-social factors from childhood onwards can greatly impact on our health as we become older. From the residential and occupational histories of 294 people aged between 63 and 78 years old they found differences in social class and gender for health that were related to the lived and working experiences of the people in the study.

Links

See Chapter 10 on the body for more discussion of sociological perspectives on the body and chronic illness.

A useful illustration of how life-course experiences and events impact on health can be found in the following extract from research by Sanders et al. (2002: 235) into the experiences of older people with painful joints brought about by osteoarthritis. What is evident here is how this interviewee clearly saw her current poor health as the outcome of the hardship that had been a defining feature of her life:

I've always done a job that involves a lot of steps and kneeling, and I've always worked because we has this old house that was condemned and you couldn't get new houses during the war, and when my husband came out of the army, we didn't have much money, he was on the buildings so … I used to do part-time work. And I done over there 15 years picking mushrooms across the road part time whilst the children were at school. And after that finished I went in different shops just working odd hours so that I was here when the children were here. Whether it was the wear and tear on the knees. But anyway, after about 20 years, I was walking on two sticks, you know during the time I was was working. (int. 8, 82 years, occupational class IV). (Sanders et al. 2002: 235)

The life course also shapes how older people come to view and experience illness. In Chapter 10 when we looked at chronic illness we noted the research of Pound et al. (1998). They found that for the older people in their study, who had survived a stroke, possible disruption to their lives was lessened by their attitudes. As a generation their experiences of historical time had been of self-denial and coping with problems life presented to them due to living through the privations of the Second World War. It was these events that forged a common stoical approach to life. For this generation, having a health problem was no different from the many other problems they expected to encounter.

Dementia

As has been stressed throughout this chapter being an older person does not automatically entail being ill. This is a popular misconception, for the majority of older people enjoy fulfilling and healthy lives. There are, however, certain conditions that do affect older people more than other sections of the population. One of these is dementia, which currently affects one in 88 of the general population, one in 20 people over 65 and one in five people over the age of 80, and is a major cause of disability in older age. Dementia refers to a variety of degenerative conditions affecting the higher functions of the brain, with memory loss being one of the most unsettling symptoms both for people with dementia and for their families. Out of the 100 different forms of dementia the most common are Alzheimer's disease, vascular dementia and dementia with Lewy bodies. In this section we shall mainly focus on Alzheimer's disease.

  Dementia demonstrates a point that was made earlier: that ageing is the result of social, biological and psychological influences. Undoubtedly, dementia has a biological basis, with a variety of causes including, for example, changes in the brain chemistry, restriction of oxygen to the brain and degeneration of nerve cells and brain tissue. It also has psychological aspects, the most notable being memory impairment. Some aspects of dementia are, however, very social in their effects and create issues for maintaining a sense of who we are and how we relate to other people. It is to these issues that we now turn to.

As a degenerative condition the effects of dementia unfold over time, beginning with disturbances in memory leading to substantial or complete memory loss in addition to physical frailty, speech impairment and emotional disturbance. This corrosion of memory and intellectual function can cause a potential destabilising of self and identity. In effect, someone can lose the memories of their life and facets of their personality that makes them what they are and this has implications for their ability to function as a social being. Much of how we communicate with others is based on how we present ourselves in conversations, for example. During such interactions what we say and how we respond to the prompts and questions of others communicates how we wish to be seen. Dementia can make this whole situation problematic. Either the person with dementia finds it difficult to engage in the expected way or the person they are interacting with is unable to adapt to the person with dementia.

People in the early stages of dementia have an awareness of the changes and transformations that are taking place in their lives as the condition begins to alter their memory and other cognitive functions. This is a difficult and worrying phase, not just because of the changes they detect in themselves, but also because of the changes in how other people react to them. Langdon et al. (2007) found that a variety of issues could cause concern for people in the early stages of dementia. For example, the actual name of the condition could cause upset. 'Dementia' sounds very similar to the word 'demented', with its implications of being 'without mind'. This could, the people in the study reported, lead to them being viewed by others as being 'short on top', 'a bit funny', or 'crackers'. Being seen negatively, or stigmatised, by others could cause unease in other ways, too. Revealing their diagnosis was fraught with risk as it was feared that other people would not really understand the condition, as this extract from a woman with dementia illustrates:

I haven't told anyone. I think they will treat me differently. I wouldn't be upset though, it depends what they know. If they have heard about it and don't understand they would treat me differently. They think it's something bad – they would scorn you and not want to come near you and fully believe you are like that. (Langdon et al. 2007: 995)

Links

See Chapter 9, section 9.2 on stigma and how social attitudes can have an adverse effect on people's sense of identity.

Ultimately, the almost complete loss of memory leads to a 'social death', where the physical body is still alive, but the self is, in many ways, no longer there. One has to take care not to see 'social death' as an absolute state. Often it can depend on the views of other people, particularly relatives and carers who, for a verity of legitimate and personal reasons, may not share an 'objective' assessment that a loved one has undergone a 'social death'. Also, as Sabat (2001) points out, for people with Alzheimer's disease personhood and the self is not completely 'wiped out'. He stresses that many aspects of some form of self continue to be present, that ignoring them is to deny that person's humanity and that as much as possible should be done to support and nurture the sense of self of someone with dementia.

Sweeting and Gilhooly (1997) found many complexities and subtleties in how carers managed their encounters and relationships with a spouse or family member with dementia. Their research uncovered various strategies that carers had developed, focusing on a combination of believing and behaving as if a loved one was socially dead. This could mean stating openly that the person with dementia might be better off if they passed away, for instance, while perhaps caring for that person on a physical rather than social or emotional level. Other carers in the survey adopted a different strategy: while accepting that the person they were caring for was socially dead their behaviour towards that person was otherwise. This entailed carrying on as much as possible with life as it had been prior to the onset of dementia. For example, making sure the person with dementia was always included in social interaction and familiar activities, such as the playing of bingo, still went ahead. A third group believed and behaved as if the person with dementia was not socially dead.

The above discussion has sought to highlight the range, extent and consequences of disease and disability among older people. It is clear that while there are specific conditions associated with the onset of old age, that many people experience an old age relatively free of such complaints. Significantly, that the consequences of disease and acute conditions may be considerably different for older people than for the younger population. Older people have a greater tendency to experience multiple pathologies, with each condition compounding the one before. Their health experiences have also to be considered within a social context where ageing is seen in negative terms and assumptions are made about the inevitability of disease and decline as part of the ageing process.

Conclusion

The main message both from this discussion and from the current research is that old age does not automatically equal infirmity, disability or poor health. Indeed, the majority of older people lead active and healthy lives. What do create issues and challenges for older people are the negative stereotypes and images attached to being old in contemporary society. Ageist attitudes still persist, whether these are expressed in the actions of private individuals or institutions.

What it means to be older in the early part of the twenty-first century is quite different from other times. Being older now can be (for those with the requisite resources) a phase in life where ambitions and life-goals can be realised. Old age does not automatically mean poverty or deprivation. The increasing numbers of older people allied with the rise of a consumerist society, through which they can express their identity and sense of self, will hopefully lead to a re-evaluation of how older people are perceived and understood.

SUMMARY POINTS

- Old age is an inevitable phase of human lives, yet can be subject to negative ageist attitudes.
- The vast majority of older people enjoy healthy active lives and it is incorrect to assume that old age automatically equals poor health.
- What it is to be old in contemporary society is changing, with many older people enjoying a 'golden age' in their lives made possible by access to consumer culture.
- The life course is a combination of historical and biographical time.
- Older people's lives are influenced by their experiences over their life course. Those with employment histories low in control and status tend to have poorer health as they age.

Case study

Joan's first memories as a very young child of five are of an air raid during the Second World War when she was growing up in Glasgow. She remembers the sound of the sirens and the deafening explosion of a bomb falling on her street. She also remembers her mother constantly telling her off for wasting anything, whether it was food, clothing or just about anything. But that was all part of the scarcity of the war years and in the rest of the 1940s when she was growing up. This culture of thrift and saving up for a rainy day made a big impression on her. These were to be values she would hold throughout her life.

In early 1961 she met Dave, who asked her to marry him a year later. Life in the sixties was a great deal more pleasurable than it had been previously. Dave and Joan managed to find themselves well paid jobs and, even though, Joan still saved and was always reluctant to buy anything she considered unnecessary, they both enjoyed themselves. Music was a particular pasttime. First it was the Beatles, and then some of the more obscure and alternative American bands as the sixties progressed. Despite her thrift, Joan had one passion: clothes. She remembered her own mum as only having one or two outfits, but now there was so much choice and each season had new styles, and there was so much more to buy than ever before.

Life carried on in this vein into the seventies. Now in their early thirties Dave and Joan began a family of their own. All went well, Dave had promotion at work and they gained a modest level of affluence. Not enough, perhaps, to regard themselves as well-off, but definitely as comfortable. Life progressed reasonably well during the eighties, but Joan and Dave noticed that the Conservative government of the day was making changes to the welfare state, and many of the sureties of state provision that they assumed would be there as they grew older were beginning to be rolled back. The ability to save and be good with money learned in her early life served Joan well, however. She made sure that enough money was put away each month in a private pension plan and other investments.

In the early 2000s both Joan and Dave retired. With their children now mature adults leading their own lives and away from home, Joan and Dave found that they had both free time and enough financial resources to do something with that time. Joan found that she could rekindle her youthful penchant for clothes and dressed very stylishly, though she always felt tentative about trying on anything that was too 'young' for her. She and Dave also began to do some travelling. They had a holiday in San Francisco. This allowed them to realise a lifetime ambition: visiting the city where so many of their favourite bands came from during the sixties.

Lately, as Joan is now in her early seventies, she's noticed that she's beginning to feel a little tired more often, and finding it much harder both to move around her house and go about in town. This is unsettling for her as she always liked to be active. She also dislikes the idea of how other people act towards her. The other day someone called her an OAP; that made her feel old. But, as she herself always points out, life is what you make it.

1   Which of the three sociological theories concerning ageing best fits this case study?
2   Identify how Joan's experiences in both biographical and historical time have influenced her life.
3   In what ways has consumerism been a part of Joan's life?
4   Why is the presentation of the body so important in contemporary society?

Taking your studies further

This chapter will have helped you understand many of the key terms, concepts, theories and debates relating to health, ageing and the life course. Listed below are journal articles and books that will provide deeper and more detailed discussions of the points raised in this chapter. You will also find what is available on the companion website. This offers downloads of relevant material, plus links to useful websites in addition to podcasts and other features.

Recommended reading

Books

Gilleard, C. and Higgs, P. (2005) *Contexts of Ageing: Class, Cohort and Community*. Cambridge: Polity.

Hepworth, M. (2000) *Stories of Ageing (Rethinking Ageing)*. Buckingham: Open University Press.

Hockey, J. and James, A. (2003) *Social Identities across the Lifecourse*. Basingstoke: Palgrave Macmillan.

Journal articles

Tulle, E. and Mooney, E. (2002) 'Moving to "age-appropriate" housing: government and self in later life', *Sociology*, 8 (36): 685–702.

On the companion website

Bond, J., Peace, S.M., Dittmann-Kohli, F. and Westerhoff, G. (2007) *Ageing in Society: European Perspectives on Gerontology*. London: Sage, Chapter 6.

SECTION 3

Contexts

12

Places of care

MAIN POINTS

- Health and social care occurs in distinct places and these places can exert influences over that care, and the quality of life for the people receiving that care.
- Many sociological theories draw attention to the problems of institutional care, which at worst can result in the loss of identity and residents becoming institutionalised.
- Recent shifts towards community care bring fresh challenges. There exist problems in defining community, plus evidence suggests that community involvement is giving way to increasing individualism.
- Informal care given by friends and family is an important feature of supporting and looking after people in the community.
- The act of caring can bring about changes in the home and in relationships between those who receive and those who give care.

KEY CONCEPTS

Organisations, bureaucracy, informal routines, surveillance, resistance, institutions, institutionalisation, community, community care, care and carers.

Introduction

All health care takes place in some spatial context or location, whether it is a hospital, an institution or the **community**. Each of these contexts brings with it a range of issues and challenges, all of which are open to sociological interpretation. This chapter will begin by looking at organisations generally and evaluate some of the major theories that attempt to understand institutions. Max Weber's classic theory of rationality and bureaucracy will be outlined, followed by Michel Foucault's views on the organisation of physical space and **surveillance**. How people subvert and manage to bend the rules will be examined next.

Where health care takes place is often decided by **social policy**, and since the introduction of the 1990 NHS and Community Care Act there has been a shift towards caring for people in the community as opposed to institutional settings. Critiques of institutional, or asylum, care will be discussed, focusing on the work of Foucault and Andrew Scull. More attention will be given to Erving Goffman's seminal work on institutionalisation and the negative effects of institutional care. Care in the community was proposed as an alternative and better form of care. However, it too is problematic. One difficulty is in trying to define what a community really is, with multiple and different uses of the concept in existence. Even if a definition can be agreed upon, there still exists a debate about whether **community care** actually changes anything and some comments will be made on how the community may just be an extension of the institution. Finally, there will be some discussion of the many issues facing carers in the community, highlighting what care involves and some of the problems facing carers.

12.1 Organisations

For many people the hospital is still the expected place or context for the provision of health care. Like many other examples of large organisations hospitals have complex bureaucracies, operate surveillance, and often involve the management of thousands of bodies. Unlike other examples of large organisations, however, they are expected to effect a positive physical or mental change in some of the people who enter through the front doors. This means that although we can use an array of sociological perspectives to understand large institutions, we must also pay attention to the differences that arise from them making life-or-death decisions about people. Attention will be given to the classic work of Weber on bureaucracy and organisations. How the physical layout of a hospital and use of surveillance affect patients and staff will be examined with reference to the work of Foucault. How people 'subvert' organisations will also be discussed.

Weber, organisations and bureaucracy

The ideas of Weber (1997, 2001) about rationality are a useful starting point. Weber, writing at the turn of the twentieth century, saw all human activity as purposeful, and in investigating **society** it is important to try and identify what meanings people attach to what they do; he termed this '*Verstehen*' or understanding. To this end he identified the following three forms of action:

1. **affective or emotional action:** action that results from an individual emotional state at a given time. If we feel happy and caring we may wish to spend longer with a patient or be more caring than we might if our mood was bad.
2. **traditional action:** we engage in certain forms of activity because we always have, to the extent that we may be unaware that we are doing it. An example of this could be the British habit of saying 'sorry' or 'cheers' in a variety of situations even though we might not actually want to apologise or wish someone good health.
3. **rational action:** this is purposeful activity where there is an intended outcome to our actions. To achieve particular ends we must also take into account what we need and what the best way possible is of reaching our intended outcome. An occupational therapist devising a treatment plan, working out what goals a client can reach and what is required to reach those goals, is an example of this.

For Weber the key to understanding the modern capitalist period was the increase of rationalisation in every aspect of life. He saw a move away from spontaneity and the outward expression of emotion, towards a society in which every aspect is governed either by rules, procedures or non-spontaneous practices, all grounded in logical, rational science. To this end he characterised mankind's condition in modernity as living in an 'iron cage'.

Weber's **analysis** of bureaucracy and organisations is distilled into what he termed an ideal type. By ideal type he does not mean what an organisation should be but rather a pure form by which to measure a particular organisation. The closer to this ideal, the more effective the organisation will be:

- *Everybody knows what they are meant to do* – everyone in an organisation should have a clear knowledge of what they are meant to do and what their responsibilities are.
- *It's clear who is in charge and who you are accountable to* – effective organisation requires effective leadership, which operates in a clear-cut, hierarchical manner.

- *Everybody follows the rules* – there are clear procedures and guidelines for whatever is undertaken within the institution.
- *Those in an organisation act with as little emotion as possible* – decisions are based on the rules and not on personal whims or desires.
- *Your position is a result of how well you can do the job, reflecting knowledge and expertise.*
- *Work and home are entirely separate spheres* – no aspect of the organisation is owned by an individual and what happens in work cannot be used for private gain.

Question

Do you recognise any of Weber's ideas in places that you have worked or had placements? If you do, did these make for efficient organisation?

Links

Chapter 2, section 2.4 discusses the ideas of Foucault further.

Physical layout, surveillance and Foucault

Every hospital is a specifically designed building, with certain features that aid its particular function. In hospitals we find rooms that are designed or designated as treatment rooms, operating theatres or consultation rooms. This may seem a useful and logical way of organising space so as to manage the complexities and functions of hospital work. Foucault, however (1970, 1979), argues that the design of architectural space is not always for some neutral utilitarian function, but often reflects power balances, authority and ways of controlling people. Prior (1993) discusses a mental health hospital built in the 1950s where there existed separate wards for Black and White people, with fewer separate facilities for Black people. This is a clear example of how prevailing 'racist' attitudes at the time were made 'concrete' in the construction of a building, with the intention to enforce a particular racist **discourse** on the people who were sent there for 'care'. Modern-day hospitals may not possess such obvious examples of control but space is managed for specific reasons. In NHS hospitals, in particular, most space is highly impersonal, with people on large open wards. Senior figures often have their own spaces that are at a distance from the rest of staff to indicate their higher power and status.

The most useful aspect of Foucault's work is on surveillance. Part of every modern organisation depends on, and subjects bodies to, surveillance. Surveillance can be seen to exist in two different forms:

Direct observation

This is where people are directly monitored or observed either by a superior or by someone in a position of authority or responsibility. Again, think of a hospital ward and how the actual space (see previous comments) is set out so that someone can monitor what is going on. In addition to making sure that the patients are receiving care and their health is not at risk, surveillance also checks that they are behaving themselves and acting in a manner that complies with the rules of the institution. There is also surveillance of staff, to make sure that they are working and performing their tasks. This may sound innocuous but Foucault maintains that it creates a form of control whereby people become compliant to forms of authority or power.

Written records

An increasing and ever-growing aspect of contemporary life is the vast amount of data, whether electronic or written, that is kept about us. Each of us accrues numerous records concerning tax, educational attainment, criminal records, career progress, health and so on. These records are a more insidious method of control, as what is written down can have a dramatic effect on areas such as career and employment. In a health care context vast amounts of information can be kept about an individual. This information could have a bearing on how well someone is cared for and treated when they have, for example, potentially stigmatising conditions such as HIV or some form of mental illness.

This outline of the various theories about organisations may give the impression that we are either like *Star Trek's* 'The Borg', living as completely perfect rational, emotionless drones working for the greater good of the collective or organisation, or that we are being constantly monitored. However, other studies, and Foucault himself, noted that people develop ways of subverting the routines and overall controls of organisations. The more sociologists studied organisations, the more they found layers of subtlety and nuance that were missing from Weber's account.

Blau and informal routines

Peter Blau (1963), for example, found that instead of workers rigidly sticking to the rules and complying with the bureaucracy, a whole host of informal working practices could develop. These informal practices, contra Weber, could actually improve the overall working of an institution. Often the complexities of what an organisation has to deal with cannot be covered by contingencies in the bureaucracy and certain flexibility is required, though never officially sanctioned. Workers may prefer these informal working practices as they can act as a relief or as a way of overcoming the effects of working for a potentially suffocating, alienating bureaucracy.

Technological changes can also have an effect on organisations and bureaucracies. The recent and massive expansion of the Internet and computer-based technologies promises to change our working and private lives.

Question

Have you encountered examples of working where informal routines were used that went against the formal rules? Do you think the informal routines produced a better, more efficient outcome than the formal rules?

12.2 Shifts in policy – the move from institutions to the community

In 1990 the NHS and Community Care Act came into being, which saw a change in the organisation of health and social care in the UK. As well as reorganising hospitals into trusts and introducing GP fundholders, the Act also brought about a shift away from caring for people in institutions to caring for people in the community. It was argued that people cared for in the community would receive a higher, more personally tailored standard of care than they would as anonymous faces within an institution. This shift in policy came about as a result of various influences that were ideological, political, or financial. Research had shown that institutional care had inherent problems that could be damaging to the health and identity of those being looked after. Writers such as Goffman, and more recently Prior, have noted that individuals can become institutionalized by their extended stay inside long-term places of care.

Institutions, or asylums as they were formerly known, have long been a feature of care within western countries and their contribution to providing effective care has been much debated. Some authors assert that by a rational progress various innovators develop new and more humane and effective techniques, while other authors note that institutions fit into the existing patterns of social control and act as agents for dominant social groups or the needs of capitalism. The writers Foucault and Scull were proponents of this view.

Foucault's critique of institutions

For Foucault the history and development of the asylum or institutional care is linked with the growth of surveillance, discipline and notions of scientific rationality from the period of **the Enlightenment** onwards. He concentrates on how the focus of the 'other' shifted away from the lepers of the Middle Ages, who had been excluded from society, to the mad in the modern period. In the medieval period, leprosy and lepers were a pariah group, the 'other' of society, routinely excluded from social acceptance and admittance to everyday life. People who were mentally ill were regarded as possessed by demons or witchcraft. Later, the emphasis on scientific rationality and scientific investigation during the Enlightenment led to increasing classification, and consequently increasing control of the population. The mad, those designated as irrational and lacking in reason, now came under particular scrutiny. Such a group posed a challenge to the new orthodoxy of rationality, and so it was they who were separated from society, this time not to leper colonies but to asylums and other places of containment (Pilgrim and Rogers 1993; Turner and Samson 1995).

Foucault highlights the use in the nineteenth century of English philosopher (1748–1832) Jeremy Bentham's Panopticon design for asylums. The Panopticon (the all-seeing eye) allows for the continual regulation and surveillance of inmates. A central tower allows observation of every cell whenever a guard or warden wishes. This gives the authorities great power to classify and control those in their charge.

Foucault is critical of what on the surface are seen as liberal and progressive forms of treatment. Figures such as William Tuke and Philippe Pinel are often credited with bringing the treatment of mentally ill people out of the Dark Ages and into the Enlightenment. Tuke founded his famous Retreat near York in 1796, where kindness and benevolence were to be the moral basis of treatment in place of the degrading, inhuman treatment that had existed before. Tuke wanted a 'desire for esteem' to replace 'the principle of fear' (Morgan et al. 1985: 152). A few years earlier, in 1792, Pinel had unchained the inmates of the Bicêtre asylum south of Paris and founded his '*treatment moral*'. For Foucault, though, these were not the humanitarian breakthroughs that they are sometimes represented as being. For him, it was the replacement of one form of control (physical) by another (moral). The mad were no longer bound with chains but were bound with strict regimes and routines backed up by moral and religious teachings, a more subtle and insidious, but just as effective, form of control (Samson 1995). The purpose of these moral controls was to turn those in the asylum into 'docile bodies': manageable, controlled entities who posed no threat to the authorities.

Scull's critique of institutions

The Marxist writer Andrew Scull (1979) takes a different position from that of Foucault in that he concentrates on the needs of capitalism, on the medical profession and on the effects of urbanisation on the development of the asylum. For him the asylum was a 'dumping ground' for those superfluous to the needs of capitalism who did not fit into the new market-led economies that developed during the nineteenth century. The poor and unemployed who were capable of working were sent to the workhouses, while those who were incapable were sent to the new asylums. Thus the removal of potentially awkward members of society allowed for the smooth accumulation of capital.

Links

Chapter 1, section 1.2 discusses Marxist ideas further.

Scull also draws attention to the opportunistic nature of the emerging medical profession. By absorbing Tuke's ideas on moral treatment into its body of scientific knowledge, the profession was able to persuade Parliament to pass the Lunatics Asylums Act and the Lunatics Act in 1845. This gave the medical profession a monopoly in the field of madness, and since they now had the power to define madness, as well as control it, they could ensure a steady clientele for their services (Pilgrim and Rogers 1993; Turner and Samson 1995). Throughout the nineteenth century there were substantial increases in the number of people inside asylums or classed as insane:

- In 1849 there were 27,000 inmates in 23 asylums.
- In 1909 there were 105,000 inmates in 97 asylums.

Both Foucault and Scull offer a view of the rise of the asylum that counters notions of a steady, value-free evolution of care for mentally ill people. For these writers, wider social and cultural forces influence and shape the development of institutions and asylums.

Goffman's critique of institutions

Whatever the origins of asylum care historically, there was a reappraisal of the effectiveness of institutions in the twentieth century, especially in the post-war period. During the 1960s the 'anti-psychiatry movement', which included writers such as R.D. Laing and Thomas Szasz, started to challenge assumptions about the nature of mental illness and its treatment, favouring a more open, patient-centred approach. Alongside this challenge to psychiatry, Goffman questioned the role of the asylum. In his seminal text *Asylums* (1961) he sought to delve beneath the surface of psychiatric institutions and expose the problems that asylum and institutional care could create. His basic premise was that the needs of the institution came before the needs of the patient and this resulted in a change of identity for the patient. In becoming institutionalised, the patient's whole personality is transformed into a shadow of its former self, and motivation, independence and individuality are lost.

Goffman begins his analysis by observing that we live in a world of institutions, whether workplaces or religious, educational or military establishments. However, there are some institutions in society that are different. These he terms 'total institutions'. In these all the normally separate parts of daily life (such as eating, sleeping or leisure activities) take place in one setting: 'He suggested that the key process – the totality – was established by collapsing the normally separate social spheres of work, home and leisure, into one monolithic social experience' (Morgan et al. 1985: 157). As a result patients inside a mental hospital can lead lives as a 'batch' – a term Goffman borrows from animal husbandry. Individuality is attacked and degraded as they become part of a homogeneous group that carries out daily tasks and functions as part of a timetabled mass.

The loss of personality and sense of self begins on admission to a mental hospital when the patient embarks on what Goffman terms a 'moral career' (see Figure 12.1), which entails the removal of the patient's sense of identity. This he terms the 'mortification of self; this is followed by the 'reorganisation of self', which sees the institution replacing what it has taken away. This process may be carried out deliberately, for example in prisons, where the prisoner has his belongings and personal clothes removed and replaced by a standard prison uniform. Or it may be less deliberate, in the case of a mentally ill patient being provided with clothing from a hospital communal clothes store. This nevertheless has a similar effect to the prison uniform for it is the removal and denial of self-expression and its replacement with clothing that suits the needs of the institution rather than the person. Goffman describes quite elegantly how the patient responds to this reorganisation of self. Goffman allows for the patient to respond in a variety of ways rather than becoming automatically institutionalised. He noted that patients can adopt various strategies for dealing with life in an institution and can develop different ways of surviving in the 'underlife' of institutions. There are five broad responses that a patient can make to life in an institution:

1   *colonisation* – the patient adapts unenthusiastically to their new situation.
2   *conversion* – the patient accepts what has happened and becomes institutionalised.
3   *withdrawal* – as far as possible all contact is minimised.
4   *intransigence* – the patient resists attempts to convert their behaviour. This resistance can be quite aggressive.
5   *playing it cool* – this adaptation maximises chances of surviving the institution with much sense of self and identity intact. It involves minimising visibility and staying out of trouble.

The 1973 film *Papillon* (French for butterfly, with its connotations of freedom) provides an example of how people respond to life in an institution. Starring Steve McQueen and Dustin Hoffman, the film deals with the lives of two prisoners in the French penal colony of Devil's Island. Throughout the movie the harsh authoritarian regime seeks to force all inmates to become compliant to its authority. In the final scene McQueen displays his opposition and *intransigence* by making a daring escape bid, while Hoffman displays his *conversion* by declining to escape, content with life in the prison. Other cinematic representations of institutionalised life can be found in *The Shawshank Redemption* and, of course, *One Flew over the Cuckoo's Nest*.

Links

See Chapter 13 for more information on community care and changes in health and social policy.

12.3 The community

The preceding section highlighted many of the problems that can arise from institutional care: dependency of clients on the institution, iatrogenic effects of care, difficulties in returning people to life outside the institution. This may imply that life and care in the community, on the other hand, is problem-free and inherently good.

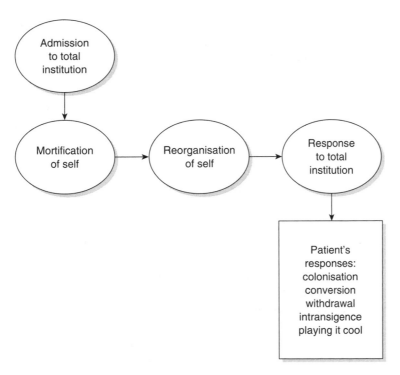

FIGURE 12.1   *Institutionalisation*

Unfortunately, much research has indicated that this is not the case. As with institutional care, there exist many problems with life in the community. GP David Widgery (1991) described returning people to the community as the 'sociological equivalent of Siberia'; the idea that people could disappear without trace and adequate support. In addition to the problems of finance and service provision there are problems of trying to understand what the term 'community' means.

What is a community?

Many British readers of this textbook may have an idea of a community as something similar to the depiction of life in popular soaps such as *EastEnders* or *Coronation Street*, where mainly working-class people live interdependent lives in a self-contained area. Occasionally the characters in these dramas may fall out, have arguments or even shoot one another, but essentially there is some form of social cohesion underpinning all interactions. If this were the case, then care in the community would make sense, as people could be returned to an area that was rich in mutual aid and neighbourly goodwill and support. This form of community was depicted in the classic research of Young and Willmott (1961) into an 'urban village' in the working-class East End of London. In the brick-built, back-to-back streets they found strong examples of mutual aid and a community that cared for its members. Dense social networks were maintained by a 'mother–daughter link' and, around this fulcrum, support for family members and neighbours was organised.

Such examples are, however, increasingly rare at the beginning of the twenty-first century. High unemployment, drug-related issues and social disintegration now blight many communities. The fabric of many areas has been altered by changes in social planning and post-war redevelopment. Chances of being part of a protective, supporting community are greatly reduced. Other trends, such as the trio of globalisation, individualisation and detraditionalisation, have been identified by Crow et al. (2002) as being inimical to the continuation of neighbourliness and community. In the US, the highly influential work of Putnam (2001) has identified that increasingly Americans are becoming detached from civic society and are less community orientated. He provides a useful metaphor to illustrate this decline in the title of his book *Bowling Alone*. In the 1950s and 1960s in America many Americans belonged to bowling leagues and regularly played and socialised as part of bowling teams. Participation in such leagues and teams has dramatically declined since then and, as Putnam argues, Americans are no longer bowling together but bowling alone.

Question

Do you think other countries are also becoming less community orientated, with people concentrating on their own lives as opposed to participating in community events?

An initial problem is trying to offer a definition of community. There have been many attempts to provide one, but the main problem is that the term covers a heterogeneous collection of interactions, situations and forms. If we look at the following shortlist of what are referred to as communities, we can see some problems:

- student community
- gay community
- business community

- Black community
- Protestant community

Question

What community/communities do you feel you belong to? What do you share in common with other people in that community or communities?

Recently, the multinational coffee chain Starbucks has been marketing its cafés as a form of community–home environment, a move that received a strong rebuke from anti-capitalist Naomi Klein: 'Starbucks pretends to sell us community, but they're selling coffee. This is a betrayal. Community is a strong and powerful idea, and I don't want it stolen from me' (BBC News 2001). What all this demonstrates is that the notion, concept and ownership of 'community' is highly complex and contested. On the above list we can find groups of people who claim to be part of a community but their reasons for claiming membership are varied. In some cases it is based on characteristics such as **race**, in others it is lifestyle, while religion or occupation may be the underlying reasons for others. In some cases these terms will reflect a distinct geographical area (for example the 'Protestant community' may refer to people of a Protestant background living in the Shankill Road in Belfast). In other cases it may not refer to a distinct location. The business community will draw membership from people living and working in a variety of settings. At other times a claim to belong to a community is made because of a choice (people choose to study at university, therefore their membership of the student community is voluntary). For some, membership is based on an ascribed characteristic (because of skin colour, for example, someone may find themselves 'automatically' belonging to a particular community).

We should consider global influences on community as well. Modern lives are increasingly infused with influences from beyond their immediate location and this too affects how people see those in their immediate surroundings. Savage *et al's* (2005) recent work on globalisation and belonging points to how the local is infused with global imaginings and meanings. Even though one may live in a particular locality, the liquidity of global flows of information and goods, the symbolic resources that globalisation provides overlay and enrich the experiences of the spatially situated practices of that local landscape. This can, for example, mean communicating with people on the Internet, or the influences on what clothes one wears or the food one eats.

Question

What examples of globalisation do you encounter in your daily life? Discuss whether or not globalisation is reordering and changing local communities and environments.

In an attempt to overcome these definitional problems we can look at some useful older work by Bell and Newby. They identified three ways in which the concept of community is used; as

1   a topographical (geographical) expression
2   a local social system: interconnection between local people and social institutions
3   a human association with no logical connection with places or local social systems. (Bell and Newby 1976)

This may sound interesting in terms of trying to crack an academic problem but when one turns to applying the conclusions to the real world, to people living in the community, then a few opposite points can be raised:

•   What community do they belong to?
•   Will someone care for ill or disabled members of the community?
•   Will that community take care of people in need?
•   Who else belongs to that community?
•   Who represents that community?

After considering these issues, another question arises: does caring for people in the community necessarily improve health and avoid the potential problems inherent in institutions? Work by Prior (1993) indicated that in many ways the problems that arise inside institutions are present in communities too. The thrust of his argument arising out of research into community care in Northern Ireland was that even though the location of care had shifted from institutions to the community, the actual substance of patients' daily lives had altered only slightly:

> For when all was said and done, they attended the same day centres as previously, they saw the same social workers, spoke to the same nurses (albeit wearing everyday clothes rather than uniforms), and usually lived with exactly the same individuals as they had done in hospital. For most people it was only the dwellings that were different. (Prior 1993: 192)

For many ex-patients, the places they were relocated to still retained many of the features of an institution, with, for example, locked doors or upper-storey windows that could only be partially opened. However, it was more than just design features of the buildings that echoed the institutions they had come from. The daily routine and the staff they saw also mimicked their experiences in an institution. Life was still lived according to timetables and they saw the same array of mental health workers. Even social events took place in the same locations as they had when the patients were in institutional care.

Question

How did you react to the preceding paragraph? What do you think of group homes – are they a break from the institution or just the institution in another format? What does this say about attempts to provide better care for those that require it?

One underlying point noted by Prior is that even though changes in discourse and treatment philosophies change practices in treating mental illness, these changes do not necessarily entail any dramatic shift in the overall circumstances of the patient. It was hoped that the movement away from care in institutions to care in the community would herald a new era of tailored, dignified treatment that broke down barriers and allowed people with mental health problems to become part of the community once more. As Prior notes, however, all that happened for many patients was a change of dwelling. This move might also be into an area that does not regard former mental health care patients as part of their particular community, nor welcome them into it.

Informal care is a combination of service and affection, provided on the basis of kinship or friendship. It is also mainly unpaid.

12.4 Care and carers

As mentioned earlier, the NHS and Community Care Act (1990) introduced a variety of changes to the organisation of health and social care. One aspect of this policy was to increase the emphasis on care taking place in a non-institutional context, and to 'firm up' arrangements for **informal care**. The Conservative government had a variety of reasons for introducing this particular piece of legislation, ranging from efforts to rein in public spending, a belief in the family as a unit of care, to, as part of their general ideology, an attempt to reduce state provision and to increase individual and family responsibility.

Links

The case study in Chapter 11 on older people provides a useful example of informal care.

The last paragraph illustrates one of the many ways in which the concept of care is used. Here it is in the context of policy, whereby a particular piece of policy lays out regulations or intentions about how care and caring for people should be carried out. But for most of us, talk of care, especially in an informal context, evokes images of emotions and feelings – though for those engaged in care work, caring is not just a state of emotionality. It involves onerous work and great physical exertion. Sometimes, care-giving informs ideas about **gender** roles, especially women's roles. The many facets of care and the way in which the concept of caring is used can make defining care difficult. That is not to say that it has not been attempted. Graham (1983) provides a useful definition of informal care. She sees care as being a combination of *service* and *affection*. Service relates to the 'doing' part of caring, including all the physical aspects such as lifting and handling; washing and bathing; or collecting messages and preparing meals. Affection relates to the 'feeling' part of caring; this includes love and compassion.

For most people informal care is provided and received on the basis of kinship or family ties (Qureshi and Walker 1989). As care can often involve intimate or physical contact, most people would like care to be provided by a family member, in this order of preference:

- spouse
- relative in lifelong joint household
- daughter
- daughter-in-law
- son
- other relative
- non-relative

Reciprocity is another factor involved in kinship care: kin have either cared for or will care for other kin.

Gender, class and care-giving

Much of the literature on care indicates that women are the prime caregivers within the family and society as a whole (Lee 1998; Malin et al. 1999). Summarising research, Twigg and Atkin (1994) point to how women are expected to care and how gender makes a difference when it comes to receiving additional support. Men find it easier to access services and are in some ways expected to put up with less than female carers. Morris (1989, cited in Parker (1993), observed that men are less able to take on the caring role. However, one must be careful to avoid the simplistic assumption that all men and all women have uniform experiences. Drawing on the 1985 General Household Survey, and following points made by Graham (1991) that **class** and race need to be taken into account, Arber and Ginn (1992) indicate that care is multidimensional, with many criss-crossing structural factors. They found quantitative and qualitative differences between men and women according to their class location. The level of physical impairment was only one factor that affected the care experience of households from different class backgrounds; other factors were their ability to access and use different material, financial and cultural resources. Middle-class households had more money available to 'lighten the load' of care. This could be, for example, by building a 'granny flat', or buying aids and adaptations. There was also evidence that middle-class households utilised social services more, and were better at obtaining desired outcomes than the working-class households in this study. There was also a class and gender difference. Working-class men were much more likely to be involved in care, looking after someone at home, than were their middle-class counterparts. Looking after someone at home was seen as more demanding, as it restricted employment and leisure opportunities.

Links

Chapter 10, section 10.5, discusses disability in more detail.

Experiences of care

The experience of care can vary from being fulfilling and satisfying to being draining and restrictive. As mentioned earlier, affection and feelings of compassion are major reasons for people taking on care work. By demonstrating affection and compassion the carer can realise a sense of purpose and achievement. For many carers, however, there are multiple problems, often to do with restriction of activity , time and money.

Tozer (1999) noted in her research on families with two or more disabled children that the parental carers reported that family life was restricted and they were sometimes left feeling isolated. Dearden and Becker (2000) identified similar findings for young carers, when they reported that for young people involved in care educational opportunities were restricted. Feelings of restriction are commonly noted in research findings. Summarising research, Twigg and Atkin (1994) observed that the problem was not so much restriction caused by carrying out care tasks, though that was important, but generalised feelings of anxiety at leaving the person being cared for on their own. Worries were expressed about safety, or about an unforeseen circumstance arising.

One of the commonest problems facing carers and the people they care for is poverty and financial hardship.

The experience of care: the home and the body

Care brings about many changes and challenges and can unsettle assumptions about two important areas of our lives: how we relate to our home and how we relate to our body. What we shall see in the following discussion is how care leads to a reordering of what home means and how carers interact with the bodies of their loved ones when they are caring for them.

First of all, let us consider and think about what is meant by 'home' as a concept, because 'home' is not just simply a building (a house, in other words) or a place where someone lives, but also an important symbolic and emotional resource. In reviewing the literature from a variety of disciplines on the concept of home, Mallett (2004) draws our attention to how 'home' offers multiple meanings. According to Mallett, home can be seen as:

- **Memory** – a place where memories reside, though not necessarily tied to a strict chronology or personal narrative. One obvious example of this is the placing of photographs around the home. Photographs in the home capture more than an image of someone, they also capture a particular historical moment or significant person in someone's life. The further one moves in time away from when the image was taken, the more it becomes a memory of that moment or person, and part of the personal narrative.
- **Family** – traditionally home and family went hand in hand, as the family home and the family house were the same thing. Currently, though, given changes in family structures and the increases in living alone this is not always the case. Especially following divorce and separation, we may have several homes.
- **Haven** – somewhere private that is apart from public life, for example the pressures of work. However, this is increasingly being challenged by the rise of home working.
- **Gender** – often home is seen as being a female place (though critically one where male authority is ultimately paramount), where women enact their required social roles of home-making and nurturing, with certain spaces in the home being gendered: for example the kitchen as a feminine space and the garage as a masculine space.

- **Identity** – homes act as a projection or idea of self and who we think we are. In choosing types of decoration, ornaments and furniture we are, in many ways, externalising and putting into objects our sense of self.

Question

Discuss the importance of place to identity. What trends, if any, can you observe in society that emphasise homes and houses as an important aspect of self?

We must, therefore, be aware that 'home' is a very complex concept and that when care comes into the equation many of the above ideas of what home is can lead to challenges and potential problems. A useful example of this can be found in the research of Angus et al. (2005). They found that the various practices and activities associated with caring could transform and disrupt a household, especially the emotional and symbolic characteristics of a home. This arises (unintentionally) out of the actions of health and social care professionals who are required to make the home more functional (for instance, to make it easier for the person who is being cared for to move about or to use the kitchen) so as to allow the cared-for person to remain in their own home. To do this often means moving furniture or putting in new pieces of equipment. Consequently, this can change how the home is perceived as the various symbolic aspects are disrupted and rearranged. In effect, the home can become a different place, which is no longer the physical and material representation of identity and self. These changes in the home may mirror the changes in the person, with the loss of self that is brought about by illness being visible in the loss of self represented by the rearrangement of the home.

Another aspect of being cared for in the home comes with the involvement of health professionals from the formal care sector. Though, health professionals bring valuable skills and experiences to the person who is being cared for, their presence signals another change for the home in a very important way: it becomes a place of work. The changes in how health and social care are organised, with ever more focus on the community, means that for health professionals the boundaries of their place of work have become increasingly fluid. They are no longer tied to a single location but instead move between multiple locations such as hospitals, community support offices, GP surgeries and people's homes. Again, this is disruptive of the symbolic qualities of home. Normally, when someone calls on someone else in their home it is for socialising, or is part of being friends, but when a health or social care professional arrives at someone's house they are not there for informal social interaction but to do their job.

Example

Mrs Robertson, aged 86, has recently returned home after an operation on a herniated disc that had been causing her some back pain for a considerable time. The operation was very successful, but it will take a few weeks for the discomfort to subside and for her to regain full mobility as she has to use a walking stick. To make life easier, her son has rearranged her living room so that she has more room to walk about and has purchased a high-backed chair to help support her back. In the kitchen, because Mrs Robertson finds it hard to bend down or stretch up to find cooking equipment or packs and cans of food, her son has placed many of these items on the kitchen work surfaces. In many respects, the actions of her son have made life considerably easier for her on a physical functional level. On an emotional level, however, these changes are causing Mrs Robertson distress and anxiety. The neat ordered home with the furniture arranged in particular ways has taken her years to achieve and acts as strong source of personal identity for her. But with everything in the living room pushed to the walls, it looks, to her, a complete mess and she finds it very embarrassing when friends and neighbours call round for a visit. The kitchen too was often a source of pride but now it just looks messy, with many objects that should be in cupboards now out in the open. All in all, she finds the changes in her home as much a problem as the problems with her back, but worst of all, seeing her home this way makes her feel old, something she does not like.

Much of the physical act of caring for someone involves close physical contact and interacting with someone's body, and research by Twigg (2006) notes that this can lead to many challenges. Often care is quite intimate in what it can involve, for example, this can mean helping someone cut their toenails or assisting them in using a toilet, or washing and dressing them. These activities may seem quite functional, in that they are necessary to maintain the hygiene and the general well-being of someone requiring care. For the person (often a partner or a close family member) who performs the care these activities, however, come with an emotional cost. In Chapter 10 on the body we saw how the body is just not a biological entity but is also important to our sense of self and to how we relate to others. Part of this involves strong social and personal norms concerning which parts of our body we permit others to see and touch. Allowing someone to touch intimate places, such as the genitals, is a very special and symbolic act denoting that we see that individual in a particular way. Thus, the touching becomes part of how we relate to someone on an emotional level, the act of touching being a bodily manifestation of the inner emotions of affection and love, for example. This relationship between emotions and the body is disrupted when the act of touching no longer takes place to demonstrate affection but to maintain the functionality of the body. Many carers report that they begin to see and relate to the body of the person they are caring for, particularly if is their partner, in a different way. The affection intimacy may be replaced with a functional intimacy. This can have an impact on the relationship between the carer and the person they are caring for, as they may no longer see that person as a sexualised human being or the person they relate to in that way.

Question

What taboos and norms surround the body in contemporary society, especially when it comes to touching and looking at the body? Is there a contradiction between the functional needs of care and the emotional needs of a relationship?

Conclusion

Providing a place to care for people who require assistance, support and someone to look after them has been, and no doubt always will be, a challenging issue for society. What we have reviewed here are various attempts to provide that care, and the, often unintentional, problems that consequently arise. Sociological perspectives on the rise of the asylum are mainly critical on various grounds. This can range from seeing asylums as a 'bricks-and-mortar' manifestation of the power of certain groups in society, or as a dumping ground for those surplus to capitalism's requirements. Sometimes it is the institutional requirements, needing to organise large groups of people to ensure that they are fed and clothed for example, which leads to an established identity being degraded and transformed into an identity that is compliant and easy to manage for an institution.

Shifts in government policy within the UK have seen increasing focus on care in the community. This can be viewed as an appealing alternative to some of the issues noted above. In reality, however, community care brings fresh challenges. The actual existence of community, in the sense of a definable entity which will offer care and support for those requiring assistance, is questionable. Various impulses and processes, such as greater emphasis on individualism, are causing a move away from civic involvement and being 'community-minded'. This brings into relief who will be doing the care work. Often, in reality, this will mean care being provided by friends and families. Though this brings its own rewards, carers can experience financial difficulties as well as disturbances in their relationship with the person for whom they are providing care.

How all these problems are to be resolved is still open to question. What this chapter clearly draws our attention to is that looking after someone and providing appropriate care is highly complex and multidimensional, in both the physical and financial resourcing of care and the demanding emotional work that accompanies informal care.

SUMMARY POINTS

- Various theories attempt to understand organisations. Weber stresses rationality and bureaucracy; Foucault emphasises surveillance and physical space; Blau notes the existence of informal routines.
- Institutional care has been strongly criticised on the grounds that institutions act as a method of social control or a 'dumping ground' for so-called undesirables.
- Goffman critiques institutions for causing institutionalisation – an assault on self and identity.
- Defining community can be hard, with definitions including places or shared characteristics such as ethnicity or class.
- Care in the community may create further problems and may not necessarily avoid the problems of institutional care.
- Providing care in the home can alter the symbolic and emotional elements of a home.
- The close contact of physical care provided by an informal carer can impinge on their affective relationship with a loved one.

Case study

Bill was admitted to Culliere Hospital twenty-five years ago diagnosed with a psychotic condition. Initially he was quite ill and had phases of believing that he could hear the thoughts of other people and that they were saying unpleasant things about him. After years of treatment and care the symptoms became manageable and their frequency declined, to the point that he no longer seems very ill any more. Over the years his role within the hospital has changed. He quite often assists with some of the group therapy sessions and has some responsibility for maintaining and tidying the art room. Bill was given that duty as he enjoys painting and is quite an accomplished watercolourist. Some of his work is hung in hospitals throughout the region. On Wednesdays and Sundays he even takes classes with some of the day patients, teaching them the basics of using watercolours. His skilled painting and control over the art room has sometimes led new members of staff to think that he is a part-time member of staff, perhaps a retired art teacher who wants to help in the hospital.

In many ways Bill feels happy and fulfilled in what he does and has expressed no desire to return to his family. However, recently the local health trust has been attempting to reduce the number of long-term patients in the hospital, with an eye to possibly closing the facility down altogether. To this end it has been decided by the hospital and social services that Bill is well enough to live in the community. This has made him feel highly anxious. He does not want to lose his art room or the chance to take classes. On three occasions now he has been taken to a halfway house to see if he would like it there. His initial impressions were all negative. There was no art room and the neighbours in the street did not look particularly friendly, some actually appearing quite hostile. To settle him in he was told that he would still see the same occupational therapist as he had in the hospital, and that it would be possible for him to continue to hold his art classes in the hospital. This reassured him slightly, but ultimately Bill really wanted to stay at Culliere. After all, for him it was home.

1 How has the stay in Culliere Hospital affected Bill?
2 Do you think moving him would help his mental health?
3 Why might the local community not welcome the siting of a halfway home in their area?
4 Where do you think people are best treated or cared for?

Taking your studies further

This chapter will have helped you understand many of the key terms, concepts, theories and debates relating to institutions and community care. Listed below are journal articles and books that will provide deeper and more detailed discussions of the points raised in this chapter. You will also find what is available on the companion website. This offers downloads of relevant material, plus links to useful websites in addition to podcasts and other features.

Recommended reading

Books

Goffman, E. (1975) *Asylums: Essays on the Social Situation of Mental Patients and Other Inmates.* Harmondsworth: Penguin.

Prior, L. (1993) *The Social Organization of Mental Illness.* London: Sage.

Twigg, J. (2006) *The Body in Health and Social Care.* Houndmills: Palgrave Macmillan.

Journal article

Angus, J., Kontos, P., Dyck, I., McKeever, P. and Poland, B. (2005) 'The personal significance of home: habitus and the experience of receiving long-term care', *Sociology of Health and Illness,* 27 (2): 161–87.

On the companion website

Little, M., Paul, K., Jordens, C.F.C. and Sayers, E-J. (2000) 'Vulnerability in the narratives of patients and their carers: studies of colorectal cancer', *Health,* 10 (4): 495–510.

13

Health care in context

MAIN POINTS

- The structures, funding and provision of health and social care are decided by government policy.
- Policy is often influenced by events, economics and political ideologies as much as meeting the health and care needs of the general public.
- Devolution has seen growing differences in health and social care policy between the various countries within the United Kingdom.
- The community and community-based services are increasingly the focus of care provision.
- Even though community-based care avoids many of the problems of institutional care, it still raises certain challenges.
- Health policy in the UK is still mainly based on public sector provision.
- Overcoming inequalities in health is a major focus of health care.

KEY CONCEPTS

Health, community, policy, devolution, carers, private, public, institutionalisation.

Introduction

The last chapter discussed various issues and challenges that have arisen in connection with care provided in institutions and in the **community**. Lately, within the UK as a whole there has been a discernible shift towards community services, as opposed to everything being provided in, let us say, a hospital or other centralised location. This shift has been driven by government policy and it is both useful and important to have an overview of how changes in government policy lead to changes 'on the ground' which affect the experiences of both those who provide care and those who receive care.

In this chapter, the focus will be on some of the issues and influences that have helped shape government policy on both community and hospital services. What should become evident is that the policy that governments enact is not always entirely made in response to the health and care needs of the population. Often, we see how events, social issues, economics and political ideologies exert a powerful effect on the shape and scope of government policy.

There are two 'complications' in discussing hospital and **community care** policies in the UK today. Prior to the 1990s wide-sweeping policy changes were quite rare and how health and social care services were organised proceeded incrementally and uniformly across all the various regions and nations of the UK. Since 1990 there has been a deep sea change in health and social care policy. First, policy changes are much more rapid than they used to be. New legislation is brought forth on a very regular basis, often in response to crises, such as concern over waiting times and the cleanliness of hospitals. Therefore, the emphasis is on themes more than on the actual details and mechanics of policy and legislation. Second, the actual political structure of the UK has changed, with Scotland, Wales and, given the hopeful progress of the peace process, Northern Ireland being devolved to greater or lesser extent from central control by Westminster. Scotland exercises the greatest devolved powers and has exclusive control over its health and social care policy. Admittedly at first the differences between Scottish and English policy were fairly minimal, but as devolution cements itself as a poltical structure the differences are becoming more noticeable, albeit still based on common themes. So one must be very careful in distinguishing between health and social care policies throughout the UK: the most noticeable differences exist between Scotland and England.

Definitions	
Public provision or public sector	Health and social care is organised and provided by the state through a network of different services at national and local level. Funding usually comes from taxation or some form of national or social insurance. This approach is common in European countries.
Private provision or private sector	Individuals are responsible for organising and purchasing their own health and social care. This achieved by taking out insurance and other polices with private for-profit companies. The extent and level of coverage are decided by what the individual can and wishes to spend. This approach is common in the United States.
Market system	Maximum efficiency, economy and performance are supposedly achieved by having either individuals or organisations competing against each other for customers or clients. The act of competition should increase responsiveness to customer needs. Margaret Thatcher's Conservative administration applied this approach to the UK NHS during the 1980s.
Third Way	A political ideology associated with the British Labour Party that stresses co-operation between private and public provision, by combining the best practices of both.

13.1 Community care

The term 'community care' is used to cover the range of policies, procedures and legislation that are concerned with the planning, funding and delivery of services for older people, people with learning and physical difficulties and illness, people with mental health problems, with HIV/AIDS, drug or alcohol problems and other progressive illnesses, and for disabled children. Any discussion of community care policies must, by necessity, encompass the policy developments in a number of fields.

There is a need to be selective when identifying the key policies – the sheer volume and range make this an enormous subject area. This chapter will aim to look at where community care policies come from, including a brief historical account of the move away from institutionalisation, the key policy milestones, particularly over the last twenty years, the aims of these policies and some of the realities for service users and their families.

Links

See Chapter 12 for more sociological perspectives on community, carers and institutionalisation.

It is important when looking at current policies to have some understanding of the nature of institutionalisation and the reasons for the move away from this pattern of service provision. In recent historical terms, any discussion of institutional care begins with the building of large institutions or hospitals during the late nineteenth century. Many were built as a means of providing care and treatment for people with mental health problems and learning disabilities or for people who were seen as being in moral danger.

We now know that people who lived in these large hospitals became institutionalised. By this we mean that all day-to-day activities were organised to cater for the needs of large numbers of people and not for the needs of individuals. Daily routines were set and people had little or no choice about the food they ate, the clothes they wore, the activities they took part in, or the people they socialised with. There was a very clear hierarchy within these institutions, with patients firmly at the bottom. Doors were often locked and people's freedom was restricted, particularly in terms of not being allowed to leave the hospital. The fact that many of these hospitals were located in the countryside added to the sense of isolation and dislocation from mainstream **society** (Means et al. 2003: 26–32).

The effect that this type of regime had on people who had been patients for a long period of time, of which there were many, was that they became dependent on the routines of the hospital. They lost the ability to make everyday decisions about their lives and became heavily dependent on the perceived safety and protection of the hospital. Many people found it difficult to form what would be seen as healthy attachments and relationships with other people and some went on to display more extreme forms of institutionalised behaviour characterised by repetitive movements, or patterns of speech.

Question

What theory have we discussed that provides sociological insights into institutionalisation?

The post-war years saw the first major policy development in the fields of health and social care following the publication of the Beveridge Report in 1942. This report signalled the beginning of a rapid expansion in the provision of health and social services. Lord Beveridge acknowledged that 'the community' had to take on a greater responsibility for the care of the more vulnerable members of society. Another key milestone in the organisation and provision of health and social care was the Royal Commission on Mental Illness and Mental Deficiency in 1957. Its report was the first official document to make mention of the term 'community care'. This document stated that the time had come for a shift to community care. This move away from hospital-based care was continued with the introduction of the Mental Health Act of 1959. Increased momentum was gained as a result of a number of high profile inquiries into the care and treatment provided within state-run hospitals, for example the Ely Hospital Inquiry of 1969. This inquiry found that people living in large institutions were not only adversely affected by being institutionalised, but also, in some instances, were treated badly and abused by the people employed to care for them.

It was not until the 1970s and early 1980s that there was significant policy development in relation to the care of older people. The Social Services Act of 1970 placed increasing emphasis on improving the structure of Local Authorities in order to facilitate the changes in service delivery that were envisaged. The aim was to keep older people out of residential care and to develop community and domiciliary supports such as day centres and home helps. In addition, there was a clear decision to enable people to enter private residential homes. This policy essentially channelled **public sector** funds into the private institutional sector while leaving the domiciliary sector chronically under-resourced. Private residential homes increased in number and in the absence of the necessary community services, older people had little choice other than the decision about which institution they might enter in the residential **private sector** (Adams et al. 1998: 54).

The Conservative government of the day proposed that a competitive market, that included the private and voluntary sectors, would inevitably provide better, cheaper services than a protected and overly bureaucratic public sector. Margaret Thatcher brought to the forefront of the community care debate concern about the cost of hospital and nursing-based care. She felt that the state should take a back seat in the provision of care for the elderly and those with mental illnesses and learning difficulties (Clarke 1994: 76–82). The 'Growing Older' White Paper was very much in line with Thatcherite policies. It identified the primary source of support for older people in the community as being informal and voluntary, relying heavily on family, friends and neighbours. This kind of informal support was viewed as irreplaceable. Therefore care *in* the community was seen as being care *by* the community (Tinker 1996: 199–207).

Question

Do you think there should be competition between various parts of the NHS, as the Conservative government in the 1990s attempted to introduce?

There was considerable opposition to this new direction of policy development as it was seen as being motivated by financial constraints and a desire to curb public spending. One of the main concerns was that care by the community effectively meant care by women, and the benefit payments that existed in no way compensated for the loss of earnings that necessarily occurred when a woman took on extra caring responsibilities. Other concerns, which continue to this day, were that community-based care was seen as a cheaper option, whereas in fact many would argue that for community care to be effective and of a high quality, it can be as expensive, if not more so, than looking after people in large institutions.

The Audit Commission Report, *Making a Reality of Community Care* (1986), was critically important in the developments that were to follow. The report stood as an objective and non-political **discourse** on the state of community care arrangements. Following on from this report, the government commissioned Sir Roy Griffiths to look at the organisation and funding for community care services. He produced a report called *Community Care: Agenda for Action*. This was an important milestone in that it strongly influenced the 1989 White Paper. Sir Roy Griffiths identified three main objectives underpinning the new community care policy. These focused on the individual user and carer in terms of meeting need, improving choice and promoting self-determination (Griffiths 1988).

The White Paper *Caring for People: Community Care In the Next Decade and Beyond* (DHSS, 1989) was published in 1989. This accepted some of the Griffiths proposals and held as centrally important the aims of increasing user choice, promoting non-institutional services and targeting services to those that needed them. In short, though Local Authorities were to retain responsibility for community care, they were to work far more closely with the private and voluntary sectors. It was also proposed that Local Authorities would be less involved in the direct provision of services and more involved in the assessment of people's needs and managing the care that was provided. in essence it was planned that they would take on more of a co-ordinating role. The White Paper was essentially the blueprint for what we recognise today as 'care management' (Means et al. 2003: 43–71).

It was envisaged that the process of these organisational changes would be extremely complex. When the National Health Service and Community Care Act was enacted in June 1990, the Conservative govgernment announced that implementation would be phased in between April 1991 and April 1993.

The way in which this piece of legislation has been implemented has evolved over the last fifteen years. In the early 1990s, those involved in the front line of assessing need (care managers and social workers) were encouraged to be innovative and to make use of formal and informal support services in the community. Many who were employed as care managers in 1993 will remember the days when therapies such as aromatherapy and reflexology were included in packages of care. However, the harsh reality of limited budgets soon impacted, and all but essential services were deemed 'wants' and not 'needs'. An essential part of the process of care management is the assessment of people's needs. Policy clearly instructs Local Authorities and practitioners to focus on individual need and not on the resources available. This remains the cornerstone of good practice but it is perhaps unavoidable that knowledge of the limited availability of local resources may have some impact on the assessments carried out (McDonald 1999: 15–16).

Since the introduction of the National Health Service and Community Care Act 1990, a range of additional legislation has been introduced, not to replace the 1990 Act but to supplement it. The first two pieces of legislation to be introduced were the Carers (Recognition and Services) Act 1995 and the Community Care Direct Payments Act 1996.

All of the legislation and policy discussed so far have applied to all parts of the UK. However, part of the manifesto of the incoming Labour government of 1997 was a commitment to Devolution. Following the referendums in Scotland and Wales in 1997, the new Scottish Parliament and Welsh Assembly met for the first time in 1999. Likewise in Northern Ireland, following the Good Friday Agreement (1998), the Northern Ireland Assembly and Executive was introduced in 1999. The consequence of this is that since 1997 different parts of the UK have developed different legislation and policy through their devolved powers, and this has led to different patterns of service provision across the UK (Sharkey 2007: 1–23).

Question

Do you think that devolution will or could bring about improvements in health and social care policy?

In Scotland, the Regulation of Care (Scotland) Act 2001 and the Community Care and Health (Scotland) Act 2002 are the two major pieces of legislation that have been introduced since devolution. These developments in legislation are underpinned by policies drawn up and implemented by the Scottish Executive. The main agenda for community care policy change in Scotland comes from the *Joint Future Agenda*. Joint Future is the lead policy on joint working between local authorities and the National Health Service in community care. Its main aim, as stated by the Executive, 'is to provide faster access to better and more joined up services, through improved joint working.' (www.scotland.gov.uk/Topics/Health/care/JointFuture).

In England, the most recent developments in community care legislation include the Community Care (Residential Accommodation) Act 1998, the Carers and Disabled Children Act 2000, the Care Standards Act 2000 and the Carers (Equal Opportunities) Act 2004. All have introduced key developments that have had a direct impact on service users, carers, service providers and regulatory and inspection bodies. More recent developments in policy have come from the Green Paper *Independence, Well-being and Choice* (DoH 2005b). This summed up the key themes in the way that the government saw the future of community care, and plans were set out for service users to be able to choose and buy the care they needed. These ideas were incorporated into a joint health and social care White Paper published in early 1996, *Our Health, Our Care, Our Say: A New Direction for Community Services* (DoH 2006). This White Paper emphasised the need for joint working between health and social care services. The main policy developments in England, as implemented by the Department of Health, come from the National Service Frameworks, which are designed to bring together health professionals, service users and carers, health service managers, partner agencies and other advocates (www.dh.gov.uk/en/Policyandguidance/organisationpolicy/integrated Care/Caretrust).

Underpinning the policy and legislative developments discussed above are certain aims and assumptions. Though on the surface they are widely held and adhered to, it is useful to look at them in a little more detail and to acknowledge some of the realities of community care as experienced by service users, carers and social care workers.

First is the belief that people would rather be cared for in their own homes. On the face of it, this is a fairly uncontroversial statement. Most people, when asked, would state that should they need assistance when they are older or if they became unwell or disabled, they would far rather receive this care from people coming to their house than have to move into residential care. Indeed social workers and care managers are often in the position of supporting families who are struggling with the reality of no longer being able to care for a relative that they promised not to 'put in a home'. The reality however can be rather different.

Case study 1

Bella lived on her own in a two-bedroomed council flat. Her only daughter lived about 200 miles away and visited once a year. Bella had always been determined that should she need assistance as she grew older, this should be provided in her own home. Her daughter was determined to uphold Bella's wishes with regard to this and was reluctant to discuss the possibility that her mother might at some point need to be cared for in a residential setting.

Bella was diagnosed with severe dementia and was disorientated with regard to time, space and people. Carers came to her house to help her to get up in the morning and dress her; to administer her medication; to prepare her food and supervise her while she ate it; to do her shopping and collect her pension; and to help her to wash and get into bed at the end of the day.

The reality of providing this level of support is that a number of agencies (private, voluntary and local authority) needed to be involved. This necessitated a high number of staff providing care and support. There was the occasional, perhaps inevitable, breakdown in communication if a carer was off sick or rotas had been changed. This meant that sometimes Bella could sit waiting for one of her meals, or need help getting in and out and of bed, and no one would turn up to assist her.

Even when services did run smoothly, Bella was confused by the amount of people, often unfamiliar due to high staff turnover, that came to her house. She became frightened and suspicious and often refused to let people in. When this happened staff spent an

increasing amount time trying to negotiate their way into the flat and therefore
had little time to spend with Bella. This
resulted in support being provided in a
very functional way with little time for
social interaction.

1 Why might Bella's daughter be
   unwilling to see Bella being cared
   for in a residential setting?
2 What changes can health and social
   care workers bring to the 'symbolic
   ordering' (see Chapter 12) of a home?

This picture is not one normally associated with the ideal of caring for people in
their own home in accordance with their and their families' wishes. This is in no way
an argument against the provision of community care through domiciliary services
but hopefully illustrates some of the complexities involved in caring for people in
their own homes. One of the key challenges then is to ensure that domiciliary services are fit for purpose and can adequately meet the needs of the most vulnerable
people (Fink 2004: 30–2).

Links

See Chapter 12 for more discussion on issues arising out of caring for people
in their own home.

Another common statement made when discussing care in the community is that,
given the choice, people would always want to move out of an institution and back
to their own home. The pitfalls of institutional living have been well documented
and were looked at briefly at the beginning of this chapter. Again though, the reality can be rather more complex. People who have lived most of their lives in an institution can find the transition to living in smaller community-based accommodation,
or even independently in their own homes, daunting and overwhelming. Their
whole identity may be tied up in the fabric of the institution that they are leaving.
They may have firmly established friendships and social networks and even jobs such
as working in the garden or the laundry. They may feel a real sense of belonging and
purpose that is hard to replace.

What is also often overlooked is the sense of safety and protection that people may
experience when living in an institution. During discussions between a patient
group from the local psychiatric hospital and a senior executive of the Health Board
in the north-east of Scotland, it emerged that the proposed removal of the stone wall
that separated the hospital from the city was viewed with horror by some patients.
They saw this wall as something that offered them protection, not a symbol of seg-
regation, as had been assumed by the powers that be.

Case study 2

Derek, Joe and Ivan had lived together in the same psychiatric hospital for approximately thirty years. They each had a long-standing diagnosis of schizophrenia, but no longer experienced any of the positive symptoms of the illness. Prior to them moving out of the hospital, it was recognised that their main support needs were the result of long-term institutionalisation rather than the illnesses that had originally caused them to be admitted to hospital.

They moved into supported accommodation in the community in 1990. Support was provided by a local supported housing project which was run by a voluntary organisation. Though keen to move into their new flat, all three experienced feelings of loss once they had moved. For a number of years after they had moved away from the hospital they continued to attend the hospital workshop five days a week, sticking to the same timetable that they had had for many years in the hospital. Through choice they continued to receive their medication from the hospital rather than the local GP. They quickly established a weekly routine of shopping, washing and collecting their benefits. In many ways, their day-to-day lives had changed little, other than perhaps the sense of pride that they now felt in being able to live in their own flat. They clearly still viewed the hospital as a place of safety and security and tried to replicate the familiar routines as far as possible in their new accommodation.

1   Why do you think that the three men in the case still feel attached to their former hospital?
2   What sociological perspectives may be useful in understanding some of the processes identified above?

Again this is in no way an argument against the ideals of community care that would say that people should be enabled to live in smaller home-like establishments that are thoroughly integrated in the community. It does highlight though the need to approach the subject with sensitivity and to avoid making simplistic assumptions. A great deal of planning and support is needed to enable service users to move towards a more independent lifestyle with greater contact with the wider community.

Alongside the aims and objectives contained in community care legislation and policy, one of the key factors in the development and delivery of services is the availability of finance to fund and develop the necessary resources. The experiences of all those in receipt of community care services and those involved in its implementation are inevitably affected by the level of funding available. Community care is one of the highest areas for revenue spending for most Local Authorities. Policy and legislation state that assessments should be *needs led* and not *resource led* but the reality is that there are insufficient resources or finances to meet the needs of all those assessed as requiring a service. Allocation criteria have been devised and employed to distribute the resources as fairly as possible. This inevitably leads to concerns about the system being overly bureaucratic, with a danger of different client groups competing against each other for their share of the pot. The challenge today for each Local Authority is to ensure that these limited resources are targeted at the most vulnerable members of society.

13.2 The concepts of health, health care and health care policy

The most well-known definition of health is that established by the World Health Organisation (WHO) in 1946. Health was then defined as 'a state of complete physical, mental and social well-being and not merely the absence of disease or infirmity' (World Health Organisation, 1992). Such a wide definition of health has been criticised as idealistic and impractical (Doll 1992) as well as for describing a state which seems to correspond more to happiness than to health (Saracci 1997). Furthermore, different commentators have urged the WHO, in recent last years, to provide a more realistic definition of health that allows the measurement and comparison of states of health and disease as well as the objectively evaluation of the effectiveness of health programmes wherever these are implemented (Saracci 1997; Bok 2004; Üstün and Jakob 2005). Nonetheless, the WHO definition had the merit of laying the foundations – more than half a century ago – for an integral approach to health care which takes into consideration the different dimensions of the human being. Largely as a result of such a holistic approach, health care is now widely regarded as the delivery of services aimed at (1) preventing and treating illness, (2) promoting, preserving and restoring mental and physical health, and (3) tackling socio-economic factors that may have a negative impact upon the individual's health. Health care policy, therefore, refers to the set of governmental strategies and initiatives related to the financing and provision of services the scope of which falls within any of these three broad areas. The rest of this section provides an overview of how health care is organised in the UK as well as of the structure of the National Health Service in Scotland.

Question

The paragraph above discussed how health should be defined as more than an absence of disease and should instead be holistic and encompassing social aspects. Reflect on this definition in light of what we have discussed throughout this book.

Health care in the UK: provision, funding and levels of expenditure

The UK health care market is dominated by the public sector, with the National Health Service (NHS) providing around 74 per cent of all health care services. **Private provision** constitutes almost 20 per cent of the UK health care system while the rest of the market is served by the voluntary sector. However, since some private and voluntary services are funded with public money, it is estimated that more than 81 per cent of the total health care provided in the UK is publicly funded (Laing and Buisson 2003; Ham 2004). The vast majority of public expenditure on health is paid for by general taxation, while the rest of the money is provided by sources such as National Insurance contributions, charges, land and property sales and tobacco duty.

Overall, levels of health care expenditure in the UK are below those of France, Germany and the Scandinavian countries. However, publicly funded health care spending is higher in Scotland than in England. For example, in 2003 Scotland had a total NHS expenditure of £1,262 per capita compared to £1,085 spent by England in the same period (Alvarez-Rosete et al. 2005). Whether it results in Scotland having better health outcomes and services than England still remains uncertain (Irvine and Ginsberg 2004).

Question

Should spending on health be increased in the UK? If so, what political issues could arise in raising taxation to fund such a rise?

Although not formally integrated within the health care market, the informal sector deserves a special mention. In fact, a considerable amount of health work is carried out every day by carers who do not form part of the health care market, like women caring for and giving support to relatives who are ill or frail (Allsop 2003). The contribution of this unpaid labour in the community to the functioning of the whole health care system is so important that the Scottish Parliament has formally acknowledged the needs of unpaid carers and promoted strategies for their support (Scottish Parliament 2002).

The NHS

Despite the importance of other sectors, the vast majority of health care in the UK is provided, as stated above, by the NHS. Before 1948, health care was provided through different sources such as private services, insurance schemes, and charities and voluntary hospitals. However, these services did not cover the health needs of large sectors of the population, such as those who were not insured workers and chronic patients who could not afford to pay for their health care, the care of whom was often left to overcrowded and poorly resourced infirmaries. In addition, hospital care was not included within insurance-based schemes, so that only primary care was provided to insured workers in return for their contributions.

The above situation was addressed in 1948 with the creation of the NHS, which was founded upon the following principles:

- *Universality and equity,* which means that all members of the UK population have the right to equitable access to NHS services regardless of income, socio-demo graphic background and health status. Therefore, with the implementation of the NHS health care was enshrined in practice as a fundamental human right to which everyone, without exception or distinction, is entitled.
- *Comprehensiveness* of the services provided. As noted above, before the creation of the NHS, insured workers had only access to primary care services in return for their contributions. However, the situation changed with the creation of the NHS, which is intended to cover all health needs of the population through a variety of services such as primary care, hospital care, and community health services.
- *Free health care* at the point of delivery, financed from general taxation. No longer should anybody be excluded from access to health care services due to their lack of financial resources.

Question

Discuss what you think about the founding principles of the NHS. Do you think they are still relevant in contemporary Britain?

While the NHS has remained a cornerstone of British society since 1948, the above principles have somehow been eroded over the last decades by the introduction of charges for some services – e.g. prescriptions, some dental treatment and spectacles – and the prioritising and rationing of resources. Besides, the NHS underwent a major reform with the implementation of the 1990 NHS and Community Care Act (Department of Health 1990). This introduced a process of decentralisation in the organisation and provision of health care whereby responsibilities traditionally considered the role of the Department of Health were transferred to lower-level authorities (Allsop 2003). The 1990 Act also created a split between budget holders or purchasers of services and health care trusts, independent organisations which provide hospital services and care in the community. The changes brought by the 1990 Act encouraged the application, to a certain extent, of market principles – like competition between providers – which were expected to result in higher-quality, transparent and accountable services offered at competitive costs.

The NHS reforms initiated by the Conservative governments have generally been consolidated by their Labour successors, which published the 2000 *NHS Plan* (Department of Health 2000), an ambitious programme to transform the NHS over the following ten years. Perhaps the most significant change in relation to previous policies is that, although maintaining the purchaser/provider split within a quasi-market context, the 2000 *NHS Plan* shifts the emphasis from competition between providers to a more collaborative, longer-term approach between purchasers and providers of health care services. It also continues to strengthen the role of management within health care settings, a factor which, coupled with the rise of consumerism and public expectations, has led to a relative decline of medical dominance within the NHS (Allsop 2003).

The NHS in Scotland

In 1999 responsibility for health was devolved to the Scottish political institutions. The Scottish Parliament has now the power to pass laws in the area of health, and the Minister for Health and Community Care within the Scottish Executive is responsible for the overall running of the health and community care services in Scotland. In 2000, the Scottish Executive Health Department – the government department designed to set health care policies as well as to manage the NHS – published *Our National Health: A plan for action, a plan for change* (Scottish Executive 2000a), the Scottish national health strategy. This document contains the Scottish Executive's plans to reform the NHS according to the principles of standard setting, public involvement and health improvement – with special emphasis on coronary heart disease, cancer, mental health and the health of children and older people (Pullen 2002).

In Scotland, the NHS provides the following services or levels of care:

- *Primary care*, which includes general practice, dentistry, optics, pharmacy and community nursing. These services are mostly delivered by *community health partnerships* which, although formally integrated within NHS boards, manage their own budget and have relatively high decision-making levels.
- *Secondary or hospital care*, provided by the NHS Boards – which own hospitals and are managed by their own boards of governors – and several Special Health Boards.
- *Tertiary care*, which consists of highly specialised services for unusual or complex clinical problems.

- *Community care* for older people, individuals with mental health problems and individuals with a learning disability is also provided by NHS Boards in partnership with local authorities.
- Public health, which involves major initiatives aimed at disease prevention as well as health promotion among the general population of Scotland. These areas are the responsibility of public health departments integrated into each NHS Board.

Health inequalities in the UK

Despite the NHS principles of comprehensiveness of care and equitable access to NHS services for all sections of the UK population, some groups appear to be significantly healthier than others. While health inequalities can be somehow associated with factors such as geography, age, **gender**, **ethnicity**, mental health status and disability, a considerable body of evidence – which will be examined below – suggests that socio-economic inequalities are the main contributor to the health divide. The first major study to investigate health differentials between social classes in the UK was commissioned by the Labour government in 1976. The study –known as the *Black Report* (Black et al. 1980) showed an overall poorer health experience amongst lower occupational groups: for example, mortality levels for unskilled manual workers were 2.5 times higher than for professional workers. The findings of the Black Report were confirmed and expanded by 'The Health Divide' (Whitehead 1987) and the *Independent Inquiry into Inequalities in Health* (Acheson et al. 1998). This inquiry, also known as the *Acheson Report*, found that the health gap in the UK had been widening since the 1970s. By the early 1990s mortality amongst unskilled workers was three times higher than for those in professional occupations. Another example is the increase in life expectancy between the late 1970s and the late 1980s, which was higher for individuals in the highest occupational groups – two years for men and women – than for those in the lowest classes – 1.4 years for men and one year for women (Hattersly 1997).

The problem of health disparities is particularly serious in Scotland. First of all, comparative studies show that health and life expectancy in Scotland – particularly among women – are poor compared to the rest of the UK and most Northern and Western European countries (Hanlon et al. 2001; Leon et al. 2001). In addition, health inequalities between socio-economic groups in Scotland have increased over the last decades (Shaw et al. 1999). A major study commissioned by the Health Promotion Policy Unit in partnership with the Public Health Institute of Scotland (Blamey et al. 2002) has reviewed the evidence in this area, providing – amongst others – the following examples of health differentials within Scotland:

- The differential in premature death rates between the 'best health' and the 'worst health' areas of Scotland increased over the 1990s (Rahman et al. 2000).

- Individuals living in the most deprived areas of Scotland are between two and three times more likely to experience lung cancer than those living in the least deprived areas (Sharp and Brewster 1999; Scottish Executive 2001a).
- The risk of dying from coronary heart disease is 2.5 times greater amongst individuals living in the most deprived areas of Scotland compared to those living in the least deprived areas (Scottish Executive 2001a).
- Since 1995, consumption of fresh fruit increased more in the least deprived areas of Scotland than in the most deprived ones (Shaw et al. 2000).

A more recent study produced by the New Policy Institute for the Joseph Rowntree Foundation shows similar findings. For example, individuals aged 35–59 living in social housing are three times more likely to have a limiting long-standing illness than owner-occupiers within the same age range, and the proportion of babies born with a low birthweight is twice as high in the most deprived areas compared to areas with below-average deprivation rates (Palmer et al. 2005). The above and other examples demonstrate that, despite certain progress in Scotland's overall health profile, substantial health inequalities still remain between different socio-economic groups.

Links

See Chapter 6 for more information on class and health inequalities.

Policy developments and strategies

Initiatives in this area during the 1980s and early 1990s put considerable emphasis on the role of health-related behaviours (Fulop et al. 1998). However, the evidence presented in the *Independent Inquiry into Inequalities in Health* (Acheson et al. 1998) showed the major impact of socio-economic factors on health inequalities. Shortly after the publication of the *Independent Inquiry* the British government published the public health White Paper *Saving Lives: Our Healthier Nation* (Department of Health 1999a). Besides broad priority areas and new targets for health improvement, the White Paper expressed the government's commitment to reducing health inequalities. This area was expanded in *Reducing Health Inequalities: An Action Report* (Department of Health 1999b), *The NHS Plan* (Department of Health 2000), and in *Tackling Health Inequalities: A Programme for Action* (Department of Health 2003), which set out the national strategy to tackle health inequalities in England over the following three years. A new White Paper was released in 2004: in *Choosing Health: Making Healthy Choices Easier* (Department of Health 2004), the government focuses on reducing and preventing unhealthy lifestyles and also outlines the increasingly important role of primary care trusts – particularly those serving deprived areas – in tackling health inequalities. In addition, it reiterates the targets and commitments contained in *Tackling Health Inequalities*. Progress towards those targets has been reviewed in *Tackling Health Inequalities: Status Report on the Programme for Action* (Department of Health 2005a). The report notes significant developments in child poverty reduction since 1997 as well as improvements in housing quality for lower socio-economic groups. Death rates from circulatory disease and cancer are other areas in which the health gap seems to be narrowing. However, although the indicators reported are promising in the long term, it is not clear whether they will be sufficient in order to meet the targets set for 2010.

Tackling health inequalities is also a major goal of the Scottish Executive's health policies. The White Paper *Towards a Healthier Scotland* (Scottish Office Department of Health 1999) set targets in relation to coronary heart disease, cancer, smoking, alcohol abuse, unwanted teenage pregnancy and dental health to reduce health inequalities between socio-economic groups by 2010. Narrowing the health gap also appears as one of the main themes of the papers *Improving Health in Scotland: The Challenge* (Scottish Executive 2003), and *Building a Better Scotland* (Scottish Executive 2004a), major initiatives that have been complemented by:

1 the Scottish Executive's anti-poverty strategy *Closing the Opportunity Gap* (Scottish Executive 2004b) which, focused on deprived communities, includes action in the areas of education, housing, employment and health;
2 *Fair to All, Personal to Each: The Next Step for the NHS Scotland* (Scottish Executive 2004c), a policy paper on NHS targets and performances which also includes tackling health inequalities as one of its priorities; and
3 *Delivering for Health 2005* (Scottish Executive 2005) a programme which – among other objectives – seeks to strengthen and enhance primary care services to achieve better health outcomes in the most deprived areas as well as to reduce health inequalities.

Question

What policies do you think are required to reduce health inequalities in society?

Conclusion

Despite the principles of free and equitable access to NHS services for all members of the population and comprehensiveness of the services provided, health inequalitiy remains a major public health problem in the UK. In past decades, the debate around such a challenging phenomenon has often been characterised by the advocacy of simple explanations (West 1998). However, a large body of evidence from research studies suggests that a combination of mutually reinforcing socio-economic factors is the driving force behind the health divide. Consequently, reducing health inequalities requires a strategical, multidimensional response which addresses the underlying determinants of such inequalities, such as poverty and social exclusion, unequal distribution of wealth and life chances, and adverse living and working conditions. Although recent policies in the UK seem to adopt a holistic approach to tackling health inequalities, it is still too early to know whether such initiatives will be sufficient to achieve higher levels of social justice and a better distribution of wealth, resources and opportunities (Bywaters 1999).

SUMMARY POINTS

- The organisation and delivery of care is shaped by government policy.
- Policy is often influenced by political ideology, events and economics.
- Over the last ten years or so there has been a substantial increase in the frequency and volume of new health and social care policies being introduced.
- Devolution within the UK has seen increasingly different policy initiatives being pursued by England and Scotland, though many commonalities still remain.
- Community care policy sought to provide care tailored to the needs of the individual and to avoid the problems of institutional care.
- The reality of community care is often different from its intentions. Finance is a major constraint in deciding the level of care and support.
- The NHS was founded to provide free and equal access to hospital care.
- Health policy across the UK currently focuses on the reduction of health inequalities.

Taking your studies further

This chapter will have helped you understand many of the key terms, concepts, theories and debates relating to health and social care policy. Listed below are journal articles and books that will provide deeper and more detailed discussions of the points raised in this chapter. You will also find what is available on the companion website. This offers downloads of relevant material, plus links to useful websites in addition to podcasts and other features.

Recommended reading

Books and chapters

Adams, R. (2002) *Social Policy for Social Work*. Basingstoke: Palgrave Macmillan.

Allsop, J. (2003) 'Health care', in P. Alcock, A. Erskine and M. May (eds), *The Student's Companion to Social Policy,* 2nd edn. Oxford: Blackwell.

Graham, H. (2000) 'The challenge of health inequalities', in H. Graham (ed.), *Understanding Health Inequalities*. Buckingham: Open University Press.

Ham, C. (2004) *Health Policy in Britain,* 5th edn. Basingstoke: Palgrave Macmillan.

Pascal, G. (2007) 'Health and health policy', in J. Baldock, N. Manning and S. Vickerstaff (eds), *Social Policy,* 3rd edn. Oxford: Oxford University Press.

Phillips, J., Ray, M. and Marshall, M. (2006) *Social Work with Older People, 4th edn*. Basingstoke: Palgrave Macmillan.

Websites

http://www.devolution.ac.uk/Policy Analysis.htm
http://www.dh.gov.uk
http://www.cymru.gov.uk
http://www.nio.gov.uk

On the companion website

Bradshaw, P. and Bradshaw, G. (2004) *Health Policy for Health Care Professionals*. London: Sage, Chapter 1.

Glossary

A

Absolute poverty: having such restricted access to food, shelter and clothing that it is life-threatening.

Ageism: a combination of a set of beliefs originating in biological variation related to the ageing process and the actions of corporate bodies and their agents, and the resulting views of ordinary people.

Agency: see Structure

Alternative medicine: any medical practice that falls outside the boundaries of conventional medicine. Some commentators use the term 'complementary medicine' to imply that non-conventional medicine can be used in conjunction with western biomedicine rather than as a radical alternative.

Analysis: making sense of data and deriving conclusions that inform a research question.

B

Biographical disruption: the destabilisation, questioning and reorganisation of identity after the onset of chronic illness.

C

Civilised body: a concept developed by Norbert Elias to denote a historical and cultural shift whereby the body is subject to increasing restraints that appear to limit the 'natural' body. The development of rules around eating manners is an example of how the body has become 'civilised'.

Class: a complex stratification of society based on access to and control of power, status and economic resources.

Clinical autonomy: the freedom of clinicians to make decisions on the basis of their professional judgement and specialist knowledge. This definition implies the downgrading of other assessments of the same situation.

Clinical gaze: belongs to a specific discourse on the body in which the body is perceived as a physical object capable of being observed, measured and treated with little or no reference to the person.

Clinical method: the process that begins with diagnosis and continues with prognosis and subsequent treatment.

Community: a contested concept in sociology that basically refers to a group of people who possess, or create, a common identity.

Community care: the range of policies, procedures and legislation that is concerned with the planning, funding and delivery of services for older people, people with learning and physical difficulties and illness, people with mental health problems, with HIV/AIDS, drug or alcohol problems and other progressive illnesses, and for disabled children.

D

Dependency theory: this claims that older people's lives are restricted by poverty and by being unable to access social and cultural resources.

Discourse: a specific way of thinking about and conceptualising a particular subject. The essence of a discourse is the language used to express thoughts. Science is an example of a discourse that rules out some kinds of explanation (for example spiritual) and only allows for others (for example, rational and evidenced 'facts').

Discrimination: acting in a way that treats people from another 'race' or ethnic group unequally.

Disengagement theory: the theory that older people relinquish their roles in society so as to minimise social disruption as they approach their final years.

Dissemination: making the results and conclusions of research known to a wider audience.

E

Embodiment: the experience of living through and with the physical body. Our experiences are essentially embodied. For example we experience pleasure and pain through the body. Feelings of happiness and sadness are as physical as they are emotional.

The Enlightenment: a body of thought developed in the eighteenth century, which challenged explanations of the world based on religious or superstitious explanations. Enlightenment thought, on the other hand, was based on a commitment to rational, secular and scientific explanations.

Ethics: guiding principles and considerations concerning the conduct of the researcher in ensuring that no harm is done to the physical and emotional well-being of those who participate in the research.

Ethnicity: is the cultural heritage and identity of a group of people.

F

Feminism: a broad concept that explains social structures as fundamentally based on inequalities between women and men. In general, feminist sociologists have challenged the traditional preoccupation of the discipline with the effects of industrialisation and the world of paid work and institutional politics. Such an approach, it is argued, has ignored the significant elements of society such as the family and gender relationships.

Functionalism: a theory of human society as a collection of inter-related substructures, the purpose of which is to sustain the over-arching structure of society. As such, functionalism provides a 'consensual' representation of society, based on, first, an agreement to sustain society as it is and, second, on shared norms and beliefs

G

Gender: the social, cultural and psychological differences between men and women.

H

Hegemonic masculinity: the dominant form of masculinity in society. Currently, this would refer to men who are healthy, wealthy, white and powerful and act in a 'macho' manner. Very few men live up to this expectation but it exerts a strong influence over both men and women.

Hysteria: a 'disease' once thought to be caused by the movement of the womb around the body but later described as a disease of the nervous system. The symptoms of hysteria have been described as weeping, fainting and a general malaise (James 1994).

I

Iatrogenesis: harm caused by doctors. In its most literal sense it refers to the harmful consequences of medical intervention. Illich also uses the concept to draw our attention to our cultural dependence on medicine and medical practitioners, such that we do not seek alternative explanations or alternative remedies for ill health.

Informal care: a combination of service and affection provided on the basis of kinship or friendship. It is mainly unpaid.

Institutional racism: the intentional or unintentional actions of a public or private body that result in people from ethnic minority backgrounds being discriminated against.

L

Life course: the increasing fluidity and fragmentation of contemporary society and reflects that old certainties of what one does at certain points in one's life are increasingly unstable.

Life cycle: a concept borrowed from natural science, implying a series of set rigid stages that humans move through in their lives.

Literature review: a systematic analysis of all published material that is of interest or relevant to the research.

M

Macro: the larger, structural aspects of society. In terms of criminal activities, this might refer to an analysis of the economic circumstances of criminals, and an analysis of law making and law enforcement, as well as of the role of the state in regulating such behaviour.

Market system: a system where maximum efficiency, economy and performance are supposedly achieved by having either individuals or organisations competing against each other for customers or clients. The act of competition is thought to increase responsiveness to customer needs. Margaret Thatcher's Conservative administration applied this approach to the UK NHS during the 1980s.

Marxism: a theory that explains social phenomena as primarily determined by the economic structure of society. Social change, it argues, is the product of changes in economic relationships. In the context of the modern period the advent of capitalism and industrialisation are seen as producing social divisions based on the ownership or non-ownership of property.

Matriarchy: see Patriarchy

The medical model of disability: a model that places a strong emphasis on seeing disability as an individual tragedy where, by a quirk of fate either genetic or accidental, someone becomes disabled and their life is, in many ways, ruined.

The medical model of health: a specific way of thinking about and explaining disease based on biological factors.

Medicalisation: a concept used to describe a tendency to explain behaviour and experiences in medical terms.

Method: the way in which actual data is gathered.

Micro: the small-scale aspects of human behaviour, for example why individuals embark on criminal activities.

N

Neo-material perspectives: these offer explanations of class and health inequality that emphasise unequal distribution of resources such as housing, income and access to education.

P

Paradigm: a systematic way of thinking.

Passing: attempts to conceal a potential stigma and prevent its disclosure.

Patriarchy: male domination in society, expressed both privately and publicly in culture, economic, politics and through physical violence. **Matriarchy** refers to a society that is female dominated. (See Chapter 1 for more on feminist theory.)

Postmodernist theories: veer away from all-embracing theories that attempt to explain all social phenomena. Instead, the emphasis is on the impossibility of uncovering the 'truth' about society. Postmodernism draws our attention to how our knowledge of the social world is constructed, and offers a critical and questioning approach to understanding the world around us. Also see **Discourse**.

Power: a subject of much debate within sociology. In the context of this discussion, the concept refers to (a) the ability to ensure that a particular point of view prevails in a disputed situation, (b) the capacity to ensure that someone acts in a certain way, and (c) the ability to stifle opposition to a particular perspective.

Prejudice: a negative attitude towards someone from another 'race' or ethnic group.

Private provision or **private sector:** the situation when individuals are responsible for organising and purchasing their own health and social care. This is achieved by taking out insurance and other polices with private for-profit companies. The extent and level of coverage are decided by what the individual can and wishes to spend. This approach is common in the United States.

Psycho-social perspectives: explanations of class and health inequality that emphasise the negative emotional experiences of living in an unequal society, particularly feelings of stress, shame and powerlessness.

Public provision or **public sector:** the situation when health and social care is organised and provided by the state through a network of different services at national and local level. Funding usually comes from taxation or some form of national or social insurance. This approach is common in European countries.

Q

Qualitative research: mainly to interview-based research that seeks to find out the meanings that people attach to their experiences and actions.

Quantitative research: mainly statistically-based research that is useful for answering research questions that focus on measuring the extent and range of particular phenomena.

R

'Race': biological differences between people based on skin colour and other physical features, though the genetic differences between races are extremely small.

Racism: the belief that one race is superior to another.

Relative poverty: having the minimum requirements of a particular society *in relation to other people in that society*.

Reproductive technology: a range of medical interventions (pharmaceutical and invasive), the purpose of which is either to promote or to prevent pregnancy.

Research question: the aspect of the social world that is to be investigated.

S

Secularisation: the acceptance of non-religious explanations of the world.

Sex: the biological differences between men and women.

The sick role: is a functionalist theory that outlines the privileges and expectations associated with being legitimately sick in contemporary society.

Social constructionism: the theory that emphasises the extent to which 'society' is actively and creatively produced by human beings.

The social model of disability: the argument that prejudicial attitudes, disabling environments and cultural barriers socially create disability.

The social model of health: the view that health is multidimensional with social factors, such as class, gender and ethnicity, influencing and patterning health and illness.

Social policy: how governments organise the meeting of the health and social needs of their population.

Socialisation: the process whereby we become aware of the values and beliefs of society.

Society: a range of external factors that influence our beliefs and behaviours.

Sociological imagination: a concept developed by C. Wright Mills, referring to a specific way of thinking about the world, characterised by a willingness to think beyond our own experiences and to challenge commonsense or obvious explanations of human society and human behaviour.

Sociology: the study of the interaction between groups and individuals in human society.

Stigma: an attribute that 'discredits', or prevents, someone's full acceptance in a particular situation.

Structure: a similar term to 'society' in so far as it draws our attention to those factors that help determine our experiences through the establishment of expected ways of behaving. The contrasting concept of **agency** means that individuals do not simply act out predetermined roles but 'interpret' those roles in a way unique to them.

Surveillance: a form of scrutiny and observation that does not necessarily depend directly on the physical proximity of the watcher and the watched. Subtle forms of surveillance are said to characterise modern society, as typified by the tendency of individuals to act in ways that they think they 'ought' to.

Symbolic interactionism: a theory of social phenomena from the perspective of its participants. An essential element of this theoretical perspective is the unique nature of the social world as made up of the actions of participants motivated by human consciousness. The meaning of human action cannot, therefore, be observed or assumed, but 'interpreted' by studying the meanings that people attach to their behaviour.

T

Theory: within sociology, this refers to attempts to provide systematic and consistent explanations of social phenomena.

Third age theory: the theory that old age is a 'golden age' where enriching and rewarding experiences are available due to freedom from the family and work commitments made possible by a consumerist society.

Third Way: is a political ideology associated with the British Labour Party that stresses co-operation between private and public provision, by combining the best practices of both.

References

Aakster, C.W. (1993) 'Concepts in alternative medicine', in A. Beattie, M. Gott, L. Jones and M. Sidell (eds), *Health and Well-being: A Reader*. London: Macmillan/Open University.

Acheson, D. (1998) *Independent Inquiry into Inequalities in Health*. London: The Stationery Office.

Acheson, D., Barker, D., Chambers, J., Marmot, H. and Whitehead, M. (1998) *Independent Inquiry into Inequalities in Health: Report to the Secretary of State for Health*. London: The Stationery Office.

Adams, R., Dominelli, L. and Payne, M. (eds) (1998) *Social Work: Themes, Issues and Critical Debates*. Basingstoke: Palgrave.

Age Concern England (2002) *Ageism: Policy Position Paper*. London: Age Concern England.

Ahmad, W.I.U. (2000) *Ethnicity, Disability and Chronic Illness*. Buckingham: Open University Press.

Allsop, J. (2003) 'Health care', in P. Alcock, A. Erskine and M. May (eds), *The Student's Companion to Social Policy,* 2nd edn. Oxford: Blackwell.

Alvarez-Rosete, A., Bevan, G., Mays, N. and Dixon, J. (2005) 'Effect of diverging policy across the NHS', *British Medical Journal,* 331: 946–50.

Angermeyer, M.C. and Matschinger, H. (1999) 'Lay beliefs about mental disorders: a comparison between the western and the eastern parts of Germany', *Social Psychiatry and Psychiatric Epidemiology*, 34 (5): 275–81.

Angus, J., Kontos, P., Dyck, I., McKeever, P. and Poland, B. (2005) 'The personal significance of home: habitus and the experience of receiving long-term home care', *Sociology of Health and Illness,* 27 (2): 161–87.

Annandale, H. and Hunt. K. (eds) (2000) *Gender Inequalities in Health*. Buckingham: Open University Press.

Arber, S.L. and Ginn, J. (1992) 'Class and caring: a neglected dimension', *Sociology*, 26 (4): 619–34.

Atkin, K., Ahmad, W.I.U., and Jones, L. (2002) 'Young South Asian deaf people and their families: negotiating relationships and identities', *Sociology of Health and Illness*, 24 (1): 21–45.

Audit Commission (1986) *Making a Reality of Community Care*. London: The Stationery Office.

Baker, S. and MacPherson, J. (2000) *Counting the Cost: Mental Health in the Media.* London: MIND.

Banks, I. (2001) 'No man's land: men, illness, and the NHS', *British Medical Journal,* 323: 1058–60.

Barnes, C., Mercer, G. and Shakespeare, T. (1999) *Exploring Disability: A Sociological Introduction.* Cambridge: Polity.

BBC News (1998) 'Health: public debate demanded on food poverty', http://news.bbc.co.uk/hi/english/health/newsid_172000/172922.stm

BBC News (2001) 'Naomi Klein: 'Know logo', http://news.bbc.co.uk/hi/english/health/newsid_1312000/1312479.stm.

Bebbington, P. (1996) 'The origins of sex differences in depressive disorder: bridging the gap', *International Review of Psychiatry,* 8: 295–332.

Beck, U. (2002) 'The cosmopolitan society and its enemies', *Theory Culture and Society,* 19: 17–44.

Becker, H. (1974) 'Labelling theory reconsidered', in P. Rock and M. McIntosh (eds), *Deviance and Social Control.* London: Tavistock.

Bell, C. and Newby, H. (1976) 'Communion, communalism, class and community action: the sources of the new urban politics', in D. Herbert and R. Johnston (eds), *Social Areas in Cities,* vol. 2. Chichester: Wiley.

Bellina, J. and Wilson, J. (1986) *The Fertility Handbook: A Positive and Practical Guide.* Harmondsworth: Penguin.

Benson, S. (1997) 'The body, health and eating disorders', in K. Woodward (ed.), *Identity and Difference.* London: SAGE.

Bernal, M. (1991) *Black Athena: Afro-Asiatic Roots of Classical Civilization: The Fabrication of Ancient Greece, 1785–1985.* Vol. 1. London: Vintage.

Bernal, M. (2001) *Black Athena Writes Back: Martin Bernal Responds to His Critics.* Durham: Duke University Press.

Berney, L., Blane, D., Smith, G.D., Gunnell, D.J., Holland, P. and Montgomery S.M. (2000) 'Socioeconomic measures in early old age as indicators of previous lifetime exposure to environmental health hazards', *Sociology of Health & Illness,* 22 (4): 415–30.

Bilton, T., Bonett, K., Jones, P., Lawson, T., Skinner, D., Stansworth, M. and Webster, A. (1996) *Introductory Sociology,* 3rd edn. London: Macmillan.

Birke, L. (1992) 'Transforming human biology', in H. Crowley and S. Himmelweit (eds), *Knowing Women: Feminism and Knowledge.* Cambridge: Polity/Open University Press.

Black, D., Morris, J., Smith, C. and Townsend, P. (1980) *Inequalities in Health: Report of a Research Working Group.* London: Department of Health and Social Security.

Blackburn, C. (1991) *Poverty and Health: Working with Families.* Milton Keynes: Open University Press.

Blackburn, R. (1998) *The Making of New World Slavery: From the Baroque to the Modern, 1492–1800.* London: Verso.

Blamey, A., Hanlon, P., Judge, K. and Muirie, J. (eds) (2002) *Health Inequalities in the New Scotland.* Glasgow: Public Health Institute of Scotland.

Blane, D., Higgs, P., Hyde, M, and Wiggins, R.D. (2004) 'Life course influences on quality of life in early old age', *Social Science & Medicine*, 58 (11): 2171–9.

Blau, P.M. (1963) *The Dynamics of Bureaucracy,* 2nd edn. Chicago: University of Chicago Press.

Boeije, H., Duijnstee, M.S.H., Grypdonck, M.H.F. and Pool, A. (2002) 'Encountering the downward phase: biographical work in people with multiple sclerosis living at home', *Social Science and Medicine*, 55: 881–93.

Bok, S. (2004) *Rethinking the WHO Definition of Health.* Working Paper Series, vol. 14, no. 7. Cambridge, MA: Harvard Center for Population and Development Studies.

Bond, J., Coleman, P. and Peace, S. (eds) (1993) *Ageing and Society: An Introduction to Social Gerontology,* 2nd edn. London: SAGE.

Bond, R. and Rosie, M. (2002) 'National identities in post-devolution Scotland'. www.institute-of-governance.org/onlinepub/bondrosie.html

Booth, C. (1902) *Life and Labour of the People in London. Final Volume. Notes on Social Influences and Conclusions.* London: Macmillan.

Bordo, S. (1990) 'Reading the slender body', in M. Jacobs, E.F. Keller and S. Shuttleworth (eds), *Body/Politics: Women and the Discourse of Science.* New York: Routledge.

Bosma, H., Marmot, M.G., Hemingway, H., Nicholson, A.C., Brunner E., and Stansfield, S.A. (1997) 'Low job control and risk of coronary heart disease in Whitehall II (prospective cohort) study', *British Medical Journal,* 314: 558–65.

Bradby, H. (1995) 'Ethnicity: not a black and white issue. A research note', *Sociology of Health & Illness,* 17 (3): 405–17.

British Medical Association (BMA)(1993) *Complementary Medicine: New Approaches to Good Practice.* Oxford: Oxford University Press.

British Medical Association (BMA) (2000) *Eating Disorders, Body Image and the Media.* London: BMJ Books.

Brown, G.W. and Harris, T. (1978) *Social Origins of Depression: A Study of Psychiatric Disorder in Women.* Cambridge: Cambridge University Press.

Bruce, S. (1999) *Sociology: A Very Short Introduction.* Oxford: Oxford University Press.

Bruhn, J.G. and Wolf, S. (1979) *The Roseto Story.* Norman: University of Oklahoma Press.

Burawoy, M. (2004) '2004 Presidental address: for public sociology', *American Sociological Review,* 70 (Feb.): 4–28.

Bury, M. (1991) 'The sociology of chronic illness: a review of research and prospects', *Sociology of Health and Illness*, 13 (4): 451–68.

Bury, M. (1997) *Health and Illness in a Changing Society.* London: Routledge.

Bury, M. (2000) 'Health, ageing and the lifecourse,' in S.J. Williams, J. Gabe and M. Calnan (eds), *Health, Medicine and Society: Key Theories, Future Agendas*. London: Routledge.

Busfield, J. (2000a) 'Introduction: rethinking the sociology of mental health', *Sociology of Mental Health and Illness*, 22: 543–88.

Busfield, J. (2000b) *Health and Health Care in Modern Britain*. Oxford: Oxford University Press.

Bytheway, B. (1995) *Ageism*. Buckingham: Open University Press.

Bywaters, P. (1999) 'Social work and health inequalities', *British Journal of Social Work*, 29: 811–16.

Carpenter, M. (2000) 'Reinforcing the pillars: rethinking gender', in H. Annandale and K. Hunt (eds), *Gender Inequalities in Health*. Buckingham: Open University Press.

Carricaburu, D. and Pierret, J. (1995) 'From biographical disruption to biographical reinforcement: the case of HIV-positive men', *Sociology of Health & Illness*, 17 (1): 65–88.

Castells, M. (1997) *The Power of Identity*. Oxford: Blackwell.

Chahal, K. (2004) *Experiencing Ethnicity: Discrimination and Service Provision*. York: YPS.

Chahal, K., and Julienne, L. (1999) *'We can't all be white!' Racist Victimisation in the UK*. York: YPS.

Charmaz, K. (1983) 'Loss of self: a fundamental form of suffering in the chronically ill', *Sociology of Health and Illness*, 5 (2): 168–95.

Clarke, J. (ed.) (1994) *A Crisis in Care? Challenges to Social Work*. London: SAGE.

Coburn, D. (2000) 'Income inequality, social cohesion and the health status of populations: the role of neo-liberalism', *Social Science and Medicine*, 51: 135–46.

Coburn, D. (2004) 'Beyond the income inequality hypothesis: class, neo-liberalism, and health inequalities', *Social Science and Medicine*, 58: 41–56.

Coker, N. (ed.) (2001) *Racism in Medicine. An Agenda for Change*. London: King's Fund.

Colman, P. (1995) *Rosie the Riveter: Women Workers on the Home Front in World War II*. New York: Crown.

Connell, R.W. (2005) *Masculinities*. Cambridge: Polity.

Coward, R. (1993) 'The myth of alternative health', in A. Beattie, M. Gott, L. Jones and M. Sidell (eds), *Health and Well-being: A Reader*. London: Macmillan/Open University Press.

Craib, I. (1997) *Classical Social Theory*. Cambridge: Polity.

Crang, M. and Cook, I. (2007) *Doing Ethnographies*. London: SAGE.

Crow, G., Allan, G. and Summers, M. (2002) 'Neither busybodies nor nobodies: managing proximity and distance in neighbourly relations', *Sociology*, 36 (2): 127–45.

Cumming, E. and Henry, W. (1961) *Growing Old: The Process of Disengagement*. New York: Basic Books.

Cunningham, A. (1994) 'Blood', in C. Seale and S. Pattison (eds), *Medical Knowledge: Doubt and Certainty*. Buckingham: Open University Press.

Dearden, C. and Becker, S. (2000) *Young Carers' Transitions into Adulthood*. York: Joseph Rowntree Foundation.

Department of Health (1990) *The NHS and Community Care Act*. London: Stationery Office.

Department of Health (1999a) *Saving Lives: Our Healthier Nation*. London: Stationery Office (Cm 4386).

Department of Health (1999b) *Reducing Health Inequalities: An Action Report*. London: Stationery Office.

Department of Health (2000) *The NHS Plan. A Plan for Investment. A Plan for Reform*. London: Stationery Office.

Department of Health (2003) *Tackling Health Inequalities: A Programme for Action*. London: Department of Health.

Department of Health (2004) *Choosing Health: Making Healthier Choices Easier*. London: Department of Health.

Department of Health (2005a) *Tackling Health Inequalities: Status Report on the Programme for Action*. London: Department of Health.

Department of Health (2005b) *Independence, Well-being and Choice*. Green Paper on Adult Social Care, London: Department of Health.

Department of Health (2006) *Our Health, Our Care, Our Say: A New Direction for Community Services*. London: Department of Health.

Department of Health and Social Security (DHSS) (1989) *Caring for People: Community Care in the Next Decade and Beyond*. London: The Stationery Office.

Dobson, B., Beardsworth, A., Keil, T. and Walker, R. (1994) *Diet, Choice and Poverty: Social, Cultural and Nutritional Aspects of Food Consumption among Low-income Families*. London: Family Policy Studies Centre.

Doll, R. (1992) 'Health and the environment in the 1990s', *American Journal of Public Health*, 82: 933–41.

Dorling, D., Mitchell, R., Shaw, M., Orford, S. and Smith, G.D. (2000) 'The ghost of Christmas past: health effects of poverty in London in 1896 and 1991', *British Medical Journal,* 321: 1547–51.

Douglas, J.D. (1967) *The Social Meanings of Suicide*. Princeton: Princeton University Press.

Doyal, L. (1979) *The Political Economy of Health*. London: Pluto.

Doyal, L. (1994) *What Makes Women Sick? The Political Economy of Health*. London: Macmillan.

Doyal, L. (2001) 'Sex, gender and health: the need for a new approach', *British Medical Journal*, 323: 1061–3.

Draper, P. (1995) *Myths about NHS and Rationing Health Care, Health Policy Network*. Banbury: National Health Service.

Durkheim, E. (1970) *Suicide: A Study in Sociology* (1897). London: Routledge & Kegan Paul.

Edwards, S.D. (1998) 'The body as object versus the body as subject: the case of disability', *Medicine, Health Care and Philosophy*, 1: 47–56.

Elias, N. (1982) *The Civilising Process Vol. 1: A History of Manners*. Oxford: Blackwell.

Emslie, C., Ridge, D., Ziebland, S. and Hunt, K. (2006) 'Men's account of depression: reconstructing or resisting hegemonic masculinity?' *Social Science and Medicine*, 62: 2246–57.

Faircloth, C.A., Boylstein, C., Rittman, M., Young, M.E. and Gubrium, J. (2004) 'Sudden illness and biographical flow in narratives of stroke recovery', *Sociology of Health & Illness*, 26 (2): 242–61.

Fairhurst, E. (1998) '"Growing old gracefully" as opposed to "mutton dressed as lamb": the social construction of recognising older women', in S. Nettleton and J. Watson (eds), *The Body in Everyday Life*. London: Routledge.

Faris, R. and Dunham, H. (1939) *Mental Disorders in Urban Areas: An Ecological Study of Schizophrenia and Other Psychoses*. Chicago: University of Chicago Press.

Featherstone, M. and Hepworth, M. (1993) 'Images of ageing', in J. Bond, P. Coleman and S. Peace (eds), *Ageing and Society: An Introduction to Social Gerontology,* 2nd edn. London: SAGE.

Fenton, A. and Charsley, K. (2000) 'Epidemiology and sociology as incommensurate games: accounts from the study of health and ethnicity', *Health,* 4 (4): 403–25.

Fenton, S. and Sadiq-Sangster, A. (1996) 'Culture, relativism and the experience of mental distress: South Asian women in Britain', *Sociology of Health and Illness,* 18 (1): 66–85.

Festinger, A., Riecken, H.W. and Schachter, S. (1956) *When Prophecy Fails*. New York: Harper & Row.

Field, D. (1992) 'Contemporary issues in relation to the elderly', in M. O'Donnell (ed.), *New Introductory Reader in Sociology*. Surrey: Nelson.

Fink, J. (2004) *Care: Personal Lives and Social Policy*. Milton Keynes: Open University Press.

Finkelstein, V. and French, S. (1993) 'Towards a psychology of disability', in J. Swain, V. Finkelstein, S. French and M. Oliver, *Disabling Barriers – Enabling Environments*. London: SAGE.

Foster, P. (1995) *Women and the Health Care Industry: An Unhealthy Relationship?* Buckingham: Open University Press.

Foucault, M. (1967) *Madness and Civilisation: A History of Insanity in the Age of Reason*. London: Tavistock.

Foucault, M. (1970) *The Order of Things: An Archaeology of the Human Sciences*. London: Tavistock.

Foucault, M. (1973) *The Birth of the Clinic: An Archaeology of Medical Perception*. London: Tavistock.

Foucault, M. (1979) *Discipline and Punish: The Birth of the Prison* Harmondsworth: Penguin.

Frank, A.W. (1995) *The Wounded Storyteller: Body, Illness and Ethics*. Chicago/London: University of Chicago Press.

Franklin, S. (1997) *Embodied Progress: A Cultural Account of Assisted Conception*. London: Routledge.

French, S. (ed.) (1994) *On Equal Terms: Working with Disabled People*. Oxford: Butterworth-Heinemann.

Fulop, N., Elston, J., Hensher, M., McKee, M. and Walters, R. (1998) 'Evaluation of the implementation of the Health of the Nation', in Department of Health (ed.), *The Health of the Nation – a Policy Assessed*. London: Stationery Office.

Giddens, A. (1991) *Modernity and Self-Identity: Self and Society in the Late Modern Age*. Cambridge: Polity.

Giddens, A. (1994) *Sociology*. Cambridge: Polity.

Giddens, A. (ed.) (1997) *Sociology: Introductory Readings*. Cambridge: Polity.

Goffman, E. (1961) *Asylums: Essays on the Social Situation of Mental Patients and Other Inmates*. Harmondsworth: Penguin.

Goffman, E. (1968) *Stigma: Notes on the Management of a Spoiled Identity*. Harmondsworth: Penguin.

Gove, W.R. (1984) 'Gender differences in mental and physical illness: the effects of fixed roles and nurturant roles', *Social Science and Medicine*, 19 (2): 77–91.

Graham, H. (1983) 'Caring: a labour of love', in J. Finch and D. Groves (eds), *A Labour of Love: Women, Work and Caring*. London: Routledge & Kegan Paul.

Graham, H. (1991) 'The concept of caring in feminist research: the case of domestic service', *Sociology,* 25(1): 61–78.

Graham, H. (1993) *Hardship and Health in Women's Lives*. New York and London: Wheatsheaf.

Green, J. and Thorogood, N. (2004) *Qualitative Methods for Health Research*. London: SAGE.

Griffiths, R. (1988) *Community Care: An Agenda for Action*. London: The Stationery Office.

Gupta, S., de Belder, A, and O'Hughes, L. (1995) 'Avoiding premature coronary deaths in Asians in Britain: spend now on prevention or pay later for treatment', *British Medical Journal,* 311: 1035–6.

Hall, P., Brockington, I.F., Levings, J. and Murphy, C. (1993) 'A comparison of responses to the mentally ill in two communities', *British Journal of Psychiatry*, 162: 99–108.

Hall, S. (2003) 'Women still on 72% of men's pay', the *Guardian*, 17 October 2003.

Ham, C. (2004) *Health Policy in Britain,* 5th edn. Basingstoke: Palgrave Macmillan.

Hanlon, P., Walsh, D., Buchanan, D., Redpath, A., Bain, M., Brewster, D., Chalmers, J., Muir, R., Smalls, M., Willis, J. and Wood, R. (2001) *Chasing the Scottish Effect. Why Scotland Needs a Step-change in Health If It Is To Catch Up with the Rest of Europe*. Glasgow: Public Health Institute of Scotland.

Hardey, M. (2002) '"The story of my illness": personal accounts of illness on the internet', *Health*, 6 (1): 31–46.

Hardley, M. (1998) *The Social Context of Health*. Buckingham: Open University Press.

Harris, R., Tobias, M., Jeffreys, M., Waldegrave, K., Karlsen, S. and Nazroo, J. (2006) 'Racism and health: the relationship between experience of racial discrimination and health in New Zealand', *Social Science and Medicine*, 63: 1428–41.

Harvey, J. (1997) 'The technological regulation of death: with reference to the technological regulation of birth', *Sociology*, 31 (4): 719–35.

Hattersly L. (1997) 'Expectation of life by social class', in F. Drever and M. Whitehead (eds), *Health Inequalities: Decennial Supplement*. London: The Stationery Office.

Hawkes, G. (1996) *A Sociology of Sex and Sexuality*. Buckingham: Open University Press.

Hewitt, P. and Warren, J. (1997) 'A self-made man', in A. Giddens (ed.), *Sociology: Introductory Readings*. Cambridge: Polity.

Hibbard, J.H. and Pope, C.R. (1986) 'Another look at sex differences in the use of medical care: illness orientation and the types of morbidities for which services are used', *Women and Health*, 11 (2): 21–36.

Higginbottom, G.M.A. (2006) '"Pressure of life": ethnicity as a mediating factor in mid-life and older people's experiences of high blood pressure', *Sociology of Health and Illness*, 28 (5): 583–610.

Hockey, J. and James, A. (2003) *Social Identities across the Life Course*. Basingstoke: Palgrave Macmillan.

Holland, S. (2004) *Alternative Femininities. Body, Age and Identity*. Oxford: Berg.

Hollingshead, A. and Redlich, F. (1953) 'Social stratification and psychiatric disorders', *American Sociological Review*, 18 (2): 163–9.

Hughes, G. (1998) 'A suitable case for treatment? Constructions of disability', in E. Saraga (ed.), *Embodying the Social: Constructions of Difference*. London: Routledge/Open University Press.

Hunter, D.J. (1994) 'From tribalism to corporatism: the managerial challenge to medical dominance', in J. Gabe, D. Kelleher and G. Williams (eds), *Challenging Medicine*. London: Routledge.

Hunter, M. (2001) 'Medical research under threat after Alder Hey scandal', *British Medical Journal*, 322 (24 February): 448.

Illich, I. (1976) *Limits to Medicine*. Harmondsworth: Penguin.

Illich, I. (1993) 'The epidemics of modern medicine', in N. Black, D. Boswell, A. Gray, S. Murphy and J. Popay (eds), *Health and Disease: A Reader*. Milton Keynes: Open University Press.

Iphofen, R. (1996) 'Coping with a "perforated life": a close study in managing the stigma of petit mal epilepsy', *Sociology*, 24 (3): 447–63.

Irvine, B. and Ginsberg, I. (2004) *England versus Scotland. Does More Money Mean Better Health?* London: Civitas.

James, M. (1994) 'Hysteria', in C. Seale and S. Pattison (eds), *Medical Knowledge: Doubt and Certainty*. Milton Keynes: Open University Press.

James, O. (1998) *Britain on the Couch: Why We're Unhappier compared with 1950, despite Being Richer – A Treatment for the Low-serotonin Society*. London: Arrow.

Jenkins, R. (2004) *Social Identity*, 2nd edn. London: Routledge.

Johnson, R. (1993) 'Attitudes just don't hang in the air: disabled people's perceptions of physiotherapists', *Physiotherapy*, 79 (9): 619–26.

Jorm, J.F. (2000) 'Mental health literacy: public knowledge and beliefs about mental disorder', *British Journal of Psychiatry*, 177: 396–401.

Judge, K., Mulligan, J.-M. and Benzeval, M. (1997) 'Income inequality and population health', *Social Science and Medicine*, 46: 567–79.

Kandrack, M., Grant., K. and Segall, A. (1991) 'Gender differences in health-related behaviour: some unanswered questions', *Social Science and Medicine,* 32 (5): 579–90.

Kangas, I. (2001) 'Making sense of depression: perceptions of melancholia in lay narratives', *Health,* 5 (1): 76–92.

Karasz, A. (2005) 'Cultural differences in conceptual models of depression', *Social Science Medicine*, 60 (7): 1625–35.

Karlsen, S. and Nazroo, J.Y. and (2002a) 'Agency and structure: the impact of ethnic identity and racism on the health of ethnic minority people', *Sociology of Health and Illness*, 24 (1): 1–20.

Karlsen. S. and Nazroo, J.Y. (2002b) 'The relationship between racial discrimination, social class and health among ethnic minority groups', *American Journal of Public Health,* 92 (4): 624–31.

Karlsen, S. and Nazroo, J. (2004) 'Fear of racism and health', *Journal of Epidemiology and Community Health,* 58: 1017–18.

Karlsen, S., Nazroo, J.Y. and Stephenson, R. (2002) 'Ethnicity, environment and health: putting ethnic inequalities in health in their place', *Social Science and Medicine,* 55 (9): 155–69.

Kirby, M., Kidd, W., Koubel, F., Barter, J., Hope, T., Kirton, A., Madry, N., Manning, P. and Triggs, K. (1997) *Sociology in Perspective*. Oxford: Heinemann.

Krieger, N., Chen, J.T., Waterman, P.D., Rehkopf, D.H. and Subramanian, S.V. (2005) 'Painting a truer picture of US socioeconomic and racial/ethnic health inequalities: the Public Health Disparities Geocoding Project', *American Journal of Public Health*, 95: 312–23.

Laing, W. and Buisson, E. (2003) *Laing's Healthcare Market Review 2003–2004*. London: Laing and Buisson.

Langdon, S.A., Eagle, A. and Warner, J. (2007) 'Making sense of dementia in the social world: A qualitative study', *Social Science & Medicine*, 64 (4): 989–1000.

Laslett, P. (1987) 'The emergence of the third age', *Ageing and Society* 7 (2): 133–60.

Laslett, P. (1989) *Fresh Map of Life: Emergence of the Third Age*. London: Weidenfeld and Nicholson.

Laslett, P. (1996) *A Fresh Map of Life: The Emergence of the Third Age*. London: Macmillan Press.

Lawler, J. (1991) *Behind the Screens: Nursing, Somatology and the Body*. London: Churchill Livingstone.

Lee, C. (1998) *Women's Health: Psychological and Social Perspectives*. London: SAGE.

Leon, D.A., Walt, G. and Gilson, L. (2001) 'Recent advances: International perspectives on health inequalities and policy', *British Medical Journal*, 322 (7286): 591–4.

Levinson, R. (1998) 'Issues at the interface of medical sociology and public health', in G. Scambler and P. Higgs, (eds) *Modernity, Medicine and Health*. London: Routledge.

London School of Economics (LSE) (2006) *The Depression Report: A New Deal for Depression and Anxiety Disorders*. London: LSE.

Lupton, D. (1994) *Medicine as Culture: Illness, Disease and the Body in Western Societies*. London: SAGE.

Lupton, D. (1996) *The Imperative of Health: Public Health and the Regulated Body*. London: SAGE.

Lutfey, K. (2005) 'On practices of "good doctoring": reconsidering the relationship between provider roles and patient adherence', *Sociology of Health & Illness*, 27 (4): 421–47.

Lynch, J., Davey-Smith, G., Kaplan, G., and House, J. (2000) 'Income inequality and mortality: importance to health of individual income, psychosocial environment, or material conditions', *British Medical Journal*, 320: 1200–4.

MacDonald, L. (1988) 'The experience of stigma: living with rectal cancer', in R. Anderson and M. Bury (eds), *Living with Chronic Illness: The Experience of Patients and their Families*. London: Unwin Hyman.

Macintyre, S., Hunt, K. and Sweeting, H. (1996) 'Gender differences in health: are things as simple as they seem?', *Social Science and Medicine*, 42: 617–24.

Macintyre, S., Ford, G. and Hunt, K. (1999) 'Do women "over-report" morbidity? Men's and women's responses to structured prompting on a standard question on long-standing illness', *Social Science and Medicine*, 48: 89–98.

MacPherson, W. (1999) *The Stephen Lawrence Inquiry: Report of an Inquiry by Sir William MacPherson of Cluny*. London: The Stationery Office.

Malin, N. (1999) *Community Care for Nurses and the Caring Professions*. Buckingham: Open University Press.

Malin, N., Manthrope, J., Race, D. and Wilmot, S. (1999) *Community Care for Nurses and the Caring Professions*. Buckingham: Open University Press.

Mallett, S. (2004) 'Understanding home: a critical review of the literature', *Sociological Review*, 52 (1): 62–89.

Marland, H. (1993) *The Art of Midwifery: Early Modern Midwives in Europe*. New York: Routledge.

Marmot, R.G. (1986) 'Social inequalities in mortality: the social environment', in R.G.Wilkinson (ed.), *Class and Health: Research and Longitudinal Data*. London:Tavistock.

Marshall, G. (1998) *Oxford Dictionary of Sociology*. Oxford: Oxford University Press.

Marsland, D. (1996) *Welfare or Welfare State: Contradictions and Dilemmas in Social Policy*. Basingstoke: Macmillan.

Martikainen, P., Stansfeld, S., Hemingway, H. and Marmot, M. (1999) 'Determinants of socioeconomic differences in physical and mental functioning', *Social Science and Medicine*, 49: 499–507.

Mayall, B. (1996) *Children, Health and the Social Order*. Buckingham: Open University Press.

McDonald, A. (1999) *Understanding Community Care. A Guide for Social Workers*. Basingstoke: Macmillan.

McKie, L. (1995) 'The art of surveillance or reasonable prevention? The case of cervical screening', *Sociology of Health and Illness*, 17 (4): 441–57.

McPherson, S. and Armstrong, D. (2006) 'Social determinants of diagnostic labels in depression', *Social Science and Medicine,* 62: 50–8.

McQuaide, M.M. (2005) 'The rise of alternative health care: a sociological account', *Social Theory and Health*, 3: 286–301.

Means, R., Richards, S. and Smith, R. (2003) *Community Care Policy and Practice,* 3rd edn. Basingstoke: Palgrave Macmillan.

Mills, C.Wright (1970) *The Sociological Imagination*. Harmondsworth: Penguin.

MIND Factsheets (1998) The *Mental Health of the African Caribbean Community in Britain*. London: MIND.

MIND Factsheets (1999) *Suicide Factsheet*. London: MIND.

MIND Factsheets (2000a) *Mental Health Statistics 1: How Common Is Mental Distress?* London: MIND.

MIND Factsheets (2000b) *The Mental Health of Irish-born People in Britain*. London: MIND.

Mitchell, R., Shaw, M. and Dorling, D. (2000) *Inequalities in Life and Death: What if Britain Were More Equal?* Bristol:The Policy Press.

Moon, G. and Gillespie, R. (1995) *Society and Health: An Introduction to Social Science for Health Professionals*. London: Routledge.

Morgan, M., Calnan, M. and Manning, N. (1985) *Sociological Approaches to Health and Medicine*. London: Croom Helm.

Morris, J. (ed.) (1989) *Able Lives: Women's Experience of Paralysis*. London: The Women's Press.

National Children's Homes (1991) *NCH Poverty and Nutrition Survey*. London: NCH.

Nazroo, J.Y. (1997) *The Health of Britain's Ethnic Minorities: Findings from a National Survey*. London: Policy Studies Institute.

Nazroo, J.Y. (1998) 'Genetic, cultural or socio-economic vulnerability? Explaining ethnic inequalities in health', *Sociology of Health and Illness*, 20: 710–30.

Nazroo, J.Y. (2001) *Ethnicity, Class and Health*. London: Policy Studies Institute.

Nazroo, J.Y. (ed.) (2006) *Health and Social Research in Multiethnic Societies*. London: Routledge.

Nazroo, J., Edwards, A. and Brown, G.W. (1998) 'Gender differences in the prevalence of depression: artefact, alternative disorders, biology or roles?' *Sociology of Health and Illness*, 20 (3): 312–30.

Nettleton, S. (1995) *The Sociology of Health and Illness*. Cambridge: Polity.

Nettleton, S. and Watson, J. (1998) *The Body in Everyday Life*. London: Routledge.

Netto, G., Gaag, S., Thanki, M., Bondi, L. and Munro, M. (2001) *A Suitable Space: Improving Counselling Services for Asian People*. York: Joseph Rowntree Foundation The Policy Press.

Noon, M. (1993) 'Racial discrimination in speculative applications: evidence from the UK's top 100 firms', *Human Resource Management Journal*, 3 (4): 35–47.

Norman, A. (1998) 'Losing your home', in M. Allott and M. Robb (eds), *Understanding Health and Social Care: An Introductory Reader*. London: SAGE/Open University Press.

O'Brien, R., Hunt, K. and Hart, G. (2005) 'It's caveman stuff, but that is to a certain extent how guys still operate', *Social Science and Medicine,* 61 (3): 503–16.

Oakley, A. (1980) *Women Confined: Towards a Sociology of Childbirth*. Oxford: Martin Robertson.

Oakley, A. (1984) *The Captured Womb: A History of the Medical Care of Pregnant Women*. Oxford: Blackwell.

Oakley, A. (1987) 'From walking wombs to test-tube babies', in M. Stanworth (ed.), *Reproductive Technologies: Gender, Motherhood and Medicine*. Cambridge: Polity.

Oakley, A. and Rajan, L. (1991) 'Social class and social support: the same or different?' *Sociology,* 25 (1): 31–59.

Oliver, M. (1990) *The Politics of Disablement*. London: Macmillan.

Oliver, M. (1993) 'Redefining disability: a challenge to the research', in J. Swain, V. Finkelstein, S. French and M. Oliver (eds), *Disabling Barriers – Enabling Environments*. London: SAGE.

ONS (Office for National Statistics) (2003) *Health Statistics Quarterly, No 20: Winter 2003*. London: The Stationery Office.

ONS (Office for National Statistics) (2004) *Focus on Social Inequalities*. London: The Stationery Office.

ONS (Office for National Statistics) (2005a) *Focus on Older People*. London: The Stationery Office.

ONS (Office for National Statistics) (2005b) *Focus on Ethnicity and Identity*. London: The Stationery Office.

ONS (Office for National Statistics) (2006a) *Focus on Gender*. London: The Stationery Office.

ONS (Office for National Statistics) (2006b) *Focus on Health*. London: The Stationery Office.

Oppenheimer, M. (1974) 'The proletarianization of the profession', in P. Halmos (ed.) (1974) *Professionalization and Social Change*, Sociological Review Monograph 2: 213–28.

Overboe, J. (1999) '"Difference in itself": validating disabled people's lived experience', *Body and Society*, 5 (4): 17–29.

Palmer, G., Carr, J. and Kenway, P. (2005) *Monitoring Poverty and Social Exclusion in Scotland 2005*. York: New Policy Institute/Joseph Rowntree Foundation.

Parker, G. (1993) *With this Body: Caring and Disability in Marriage*. Buckingham: Open University Press.

Peterson, A. (1997) 'Risk, governance and the new public health', in A. Peterson and R. Bunton (eds), *Foucault: Health and Medicine*. London: Routledge.

Phillips, T. and Phillips, M. (1999) *Windrush: The Irresistible Rise of Multi-racial Britain*. London: HarperCollins.

Philo, G. (ed.) (1996) *Media and Mental Distress*. London: Longman.

Picardie, R. (1993) *Before I Say Goodbye*. London: Penguin.

Pilgrim, D. and Rogers, A. (1993) *A Sociology of Mental Health and Illness*. Buckingham: Open University Press.

Pilgrim, D. and Rogers, A. (1994) 'Something old, something new … sociology and the organisation of psychiatry', *Sociology*, 28 (2): 521–38.

Porter, M. (1990) 'Professional–client relationships and women's reproductive health care', in S. Cunningham-Burley and N. McKeganey (eds), *Readings in Medical Sociology*. London: Tavistock.

Porter, S. (1993) 'Changing influence of occupational sociology', *British Journal of Nursing*, 2 (22): 1113–18.

Pound, P., Gompertz, P. and Ebrahim, S. (1998) 'Illness in the context: the case of stroke', *Sociology of Health and Illness*, 20 (4): 489–506.

Pound, P., Britten, N., Morgan, M., Yardley, L., Pope, C., Daker-White, G. and Campbell, R. (2005) 'Resisting medicines: a synthesis of qualitative studies of medicine taking', *Social Science and Medicine*, 61: 133–55.

Prior, L. (1993) *The Social Organization of Mental Illness*. London: SAGE.

Prior, P. (1995) 'Surviving psychiatric institutional: a case study', *Sociology of Health and Illness*, 17 (5): 651–67.

Pullen, I. (2002) 'The Scottish scene', *Psychiatric Bulletin*, 26: 86–7.

Putnam, R. (2000) *Bowling Alone: The Collapse and Revival of American Community*. New York: Simon & Schuster.

Qureshi, H. and Walker, A. (1989) *The Caring Relationship: Elderly People and their Families*. Basingstoke: Macmillan.

Radia, K. (1996) *Ignored, Silenced, Neglected: Housing and Mental Health Care Needs of Asian People*. York: York Publication Services for the Joseph Rowntree Foundation.

Rahman, M., Palmer, G., Kenway, P. and Howarth, C. (2000) *Monitoring Poverty and Social Exclusion*. London: New Policy Institute.

Ramazanaglu, C. (1989) *Feminism and the Contradictions of Oppression*. London: Routledge.

Reissman, L. (1992) 'Women and medicalisation: a new perspective', in L. McDowell and R. Pringle (eds), *Defining Women: Social Institutions and Gender Divisions*. Cambridge: Polity Press/Open University.

Robinson, I. (1988) *Multiple Sclerosis*. London: Routledge.

Rose, S. (2005) *Lifelines: Life beyond the Gene*. London: Vintage.

Rosenhan, D.L. (1973) 'On being sane in insane places', *Science*, 179: 250–8.

Roughhead, W. (2000) 'The body snatchers', (1921), in B.D. Osborne and R. Armstrong (eds), *Wicked Men and Fools: A Scottish Crime Anthology*. Edinburgh: Birlinn.

Sabat, S.R. (2001) *The Experience of Alzheimer's Disease*. Oxford: Blackwell.

Saks, M. (ed.), (1992) *Alternative Medicine in Britain*. Oxford: Clarendon Press.

Saks, M. (1994) 'The alternatives to medicine', in J. Gabe, D. Kelleher and G. Williams (eds), *Challenging Medicine*. London: Routledge.

Saks, M. (1998) 'Medicine and complementary medicine', in G. Scambler and P. Higgs (eds), *Modernity, Medicine and Health: Medical Sociology towards 2000*. London: Routledge.

Samson, C. (1995) 'Madness and psychiatry', in B. Turner with C. Samson, *Medical Power and Social Knowledge*. London: SAGE.

Sanders, C., Donovan, J. and Dieppe, P. (2002) 'The significance and consequences of having painful and disabled joints in older age: co-existing accounts of normal and disrupted biographies', *Sociology of Health and Illness,* 24 (2): 227–53.

Saracci, R. (1997) 'The world health organisation needs to reconsider its definition of health', *British Medical Journal*, 314: 1409.

Savage, M., Bagnall, G. and Longhurst, B. (2005) *Globalisation and Belonging*, London: SAGE.

Scheff, T (1966) *Being Mentally Ill: A Sociology Theory*. Chicago, IL: Aldine.

Schnittker, J. (2005) 'Chronic illness and depressive symptoms', *Social Science and Medicine,* 60: 13–23.

Scottish Executive (1999a) *Health in Scotland*. Edinburgh: Scottish Executive.

Scottish Executive (1999b) *Scottish Crime Survey*. Edinburgh: Scottish Executive.

Scottish Executive (2000) *Our National Health: A Plan for Action, a Plan for Change*. Edinburgh: Scottish Executive.

Scottish Executive (2001a) *Health in Scotland 2000. Report of the Chief Medical Officer for Scotland*. Edinburgh: The Stationery Office.

Scottish Executive (2001b) *Scottish Household Survey, Bulletin No. 5*. Edinburgh: Scottish Executive.

Scottish Executive (2003) *Improving Health in Scotland: The Challenge*. Edinburgh: The Stationery Office.

Scottish Executive (2004a) *Building a Better Scotland: Spending Proposals 2005–2008: Enterprise, Opportunity, Fairness: Technical Notes*. Edinburgh: Scottish Executive.

Scottish Executive (2004b) *Closing the Opportunity Gap*. Edinburgh: Scottish Executive.

Scottish Executive (2004c) *Fair To All, Personal To Each: The Next Step for the NHS Scotland*. Edinburgh: Scottish Executive.

Scottish Executive (2005) *Delivering for Health 2005*. Edinburgh: Scottish Executive.

Scottish Office Department of Health (1999) *Towards a Healthier Scotland. A White Paper on Health*. Edinburgh: The Stationery Office.

Scottish Parliament (2002) *The Community Care and Health (Scotland) Act 2002*. Edinburgh: The Stationery Office.

Scull, A. (1979) *Museums of Madness: The Social Organization of Insanity in Nineteenth Century England*. London: Allen Lane.

Seale, C. (1998) 'Normal/pathological', in C. Jenks (ed.), *Core Sociological Dichotomies*. London: SAGE.

Seale, C. (2005) 'New directions for critical internet health studies: representing cancer experiences on the web', *Sociology of Health and Illness, 27* (4): 515–40.

Seale, C. and Pattison, S. (1994) *Medical Knowledge: Doubt and Certainty*. Milton Keynes: Open University Press.

Sharkey, P. (2007) *The Essentials of Community Care*. Basingstoke: Palgrave Macmillan.

Sharma, U. (1992) *Complementary Medicine Today: Practitioners and Patients*. London: Routledge.

Sharp, L. and Brewster, D. (1999) 'The epidemiology of lung cancer in Scotland: a review of trends in incidence, survival and mortality and prospects for prevention', *Health Bulletin*, 57 (5): 318–31.

Shaw, M., Dorling, D., Gordon D. and Davey-Smith, G. (1999) *The Widening Gap: Health Inequalities and Policy in Britain*. Bristol: The Policy Press.

Shaw, A., McMunn, A. and Field, J. (eds) (2000) *The Scottish Health Survey 1998. A Survey Carried Out on behalf of the Scottish Executive Health Department*. Edinburgh: Scottish Executive.

Shilling, C. (1993) *The Body and Social Theory*. London: SAGE.

Shilling, C. (1997) 'The body', in K. Woodward (ed.), *The Politics of Identity*. London: SAGE/Open University Press.

Singer, E. (1974) 'Premature social ageing: the social psychological consequences of a chronic illness', *Social Science and Medicine*, 8: 143–51.

Smaje C. (1995) *Health, 'Race' and Ethnicity: Making Sense of the Evidence*. London: Kings Fund Institute.

Smaje, C. (1996) 'The ethnic patterning of health: new directions for theory and research', *Sociology of Health and Illness*, 18 (2): 139–71.

Smart, C. (1996) 'Deconstructing motherhood', in E. Bortolaia Silva (ed.), *Good Enough Mothering? Feminist Perspectives on Lone Motherhood*. London: Routledge.

Smith, G., Shaw, M., Mitchell, R., Dorling, D. and Gordon, D. (2000) 'Inequalities in health continue to grow despite government's pledges', *British Medical Journal*, 320: 582.

SPIU (Scottish Poverty Information Unit) (1997) *Defining Poverty*. http://spiu.gcal.ac.uk/briefing1.html. Glasgow: Glasgow Caledonian University.

SPIU (Scottish Poverty Information Unit) (1998) *Briefing 7: Disability and Poverty – December 1998*. Glasgow: Glasgow Caledonian University.

SPIU (Scottish Poverty Information Unit) (2002) *Poverty in Scotland*. Glasgow: Glasgow Caledonian University.

Stacey, M. (1988) *The Sociology of Health and Healing*. London: Routledge.

Stalker, K. and Jones, C. (1998) 'Normalization and critical disability theory', in D. Jones, S.E.E. Blair, T. Hartery and R.K. Jones (eds), *Sociology and Occupational Therapy*. Edinburgh: Churchill Livingstone.

Star, S. (1955) 'The public's idea about mental illness'. Paper presented at the National Association for Mental Health Meeting, Chicago, IL, November.

Stimson, G. and Webb, B. (1975) *Going to See the Doctor: the Consultation Process in General Practice*. London: Routledge & Kegan Paul.

Strauss, A.L. (1987) *Qualitative Analysis for Social Scientists*. Cambridge: Cambridge University Press.

Swain, J., Finkelstein V., French S. and Oliver M. (eds) (1993) *Disabling Barriers – Enabling Environments*. London: SAGE.

Sweeting, H. and Gilhooly, M. (1997) 'Dementia and the phenomenon of social death', *Sociology of Health and Illness*, 19 (1): 93–117.

Taylor, S. (1989) *Suicide*. London: Longman.

Taylor, S. (1990) 'Beyond Durkheim: sociology and suicide', *Social Studies Review*, 6 (2): 70–4.

Tinker, A. (1996) *Older People in Modern Society*. Harlow: Longman.

Tozer, R. (1999) *Supporting Families with Two or More Severely Disabled Children*. York: Joseph Rowntree Foundation.

Turner, B.S. (1994) *Medical Power and Social Knowledge*. London: SAGE.

Turner, B. with Samson, C. (1995) *Medical Power and Social Knowledge*. London: SAGE.

Twigg, J. (2006) *The Body in Health and Social Care*. Basingstoke: Palgrave Macmillan.

Twigg, J. (2007) 'Clothing, age and the body: a critical review', *Ageing and Society*, 27: 285–305.

Twigg, J. and Atkin, K. (1994) *Carers Perceived: Policy and Practice in Informal Care*. Buckingham: Open University Press.

United Nations (2005) *Demographic Yearbook 2002*. New York: United Nations.

Üstün, B. and Jakob, R. (2005) 'Calling a spade a spade: meaningful definitions of health conditions', *Bulletin of the World Health Organisation*, 83: 802.

Wade, D.T. (2001) 'Ethical issues in the diagnosis of Permanent Vegetative State', *British Medical Journal,* 322 (10 February): 352–4.

Warnock, M. (1985) *A Question of Life*. Oxford: Blackwell.

Watson, J. (2000) *Male Bodies: Health, Culture, and Identity*. London: Taylor & Francis.

Weber, M. (1997) *Theory of Social and Economic Organization*. London: Free Press.

Weber, M. (2001) *The Protestant Work Ethic and the Spirit of Capitalism*. London: Routledge.

Wendell, S. (1996) *The Rejected Body*. London: Routledge.

West, P. (1998) *Perspectives on Health Inequalities: The Need for a Lifecourse Approach.* Glasgow: Medical Research Council Social and Public Health Sciences Unit, University of Glasgow.

West, R. (1993) 'Alternative medicine: prospects and speculation', in N. Black, D. Boswell, A. Gray, S. Murphy and J. Popay (eds), *Health and Disease: A Reader.* Milton Keynes: Open University Press.

Whitehead, S.M. (1987) 'The health divide', in P. Townsend, M. Whitehead and N. Davidson (eds), *Inequalities in Health: The Black Report and the Health Divide.* London: Penguin.

Whitehead, S.M. (2002) *Men and Masculinities: Key Themes and New Directions.* Cambridge: Polity.

Widgery, D. (1991) *Some Lives! A GP's East End*. London: Simon & Schuster.

Wiles, R., Ashburn, A., Payne, S. and Murphy, C. (2004) 'Discharge from physiotherapy following stroke: the management of disappointment', *Social Science and Medicine*, 59: 1263–73.

Wilkinson, R. (1996) *Unhealthy Societies: The Afflictions of Inequality*. London: Routledge.

Williams, B. and Barlow, J.H. (1998) 'Falling out with my shadow: lay perceptions of the body in the context of arthritis', in J. Watson and S. Nettleton (eds), *The Body in Everyday Life*. London: Routledge.

Williams, S.J. (2000) 'Chronic illness as biographical disruption or biographical disruption as chronic illness? Reflections on a core concept', *Sociology of Health and Illness*, 22 (1): 40–67.

Williams, S.J. (2003) *Medicine and the Body*. London: SAGE.

Williams, S.J. and Bendelow, G. (1998) 'In search of the "missing body": pain, suffering and the (post) modern condition', in G. Scambler, and P. Higgs (eds), *Modernity, Medicine and Health*. London: Routledge.

Witz, A. (1992) *Professions and Patriarchy*. London: Routledge.

Wogan, P. (2004) 'Deep hanging out: reflections on fieldwork and multisided Andean ethnography', *Identities: Global Studies in Culture and Power* 11: 129–39.

World Health Organisation (1980) *International Classification of Impairments, Disabilities and Handicaps*. Geneva: WHO.

World Health Organisation (1992) *Basic Documents,* 39th edn. Geneva: WHO.

Young, M. and Willmott, P. (1961) *Family and Kinship in East London*. Harmondsworth: Penguin.

Yuill, C. (2005) 'Marx: capitalism, alienation and health', *Social Theory and Health,* (3): 126–43.

Yuill, C. (2007) 'The body as weapon: Bobby Sands and the Republican hunger strikes', *Sociological Research Online,* 12 (2). www. socresonline.org.uk/12/2/yuill. html

Zsembik, B.A. and Fennell, D. (2005) 'Ethnic variation in health and the determinants of health among Latinos', *Social Science and Medicine,* 61 (11): 53–63.

Index